Mutation-specific therapies in cystic fibrosis

UNI-MED

UNI-MED Verlag AG
Bremen - London - Boston

Tümmler, Burkhard:
Mutation-specific therapies in cystic fibrosis/Burkhard Tümmler.-
2nd edition - Bremen: UNI-MED, 2022
(UNI-MED SCIENCE)
ISBN 978-3-8374-1630-5

Printed in Europe

MEDICINE - STATE OF THE ART

UNI-MED Verlag AG, one of the leading medical publishing companies in Germany, presents its highly successful series of scientific textbooks, covering all medical subjects. The authors are specialists in their fields and present the topics precisely, comprehensively, and with the facility of quick reference in mind. The books will be most useful for all doctors who wish to keep up to date with the latest developments in medicine.

The publisher would like to thank the company Vertex Pharmaceuticals (Germany) for supporting the production of this edition. The publisher assures that the industry partner could not influence the content of the book in any way, especially not therapy recommendations.

Preface and acknowledgements 2nd edition

Cystic fibrosis is a severe ion channel disease of autosomal recessive inheritance that is caused by mutations in the Cystic Fibrosis Transmembrane Conductance Regulator (CFTR) gene. Thanks to continuously improved symptomatic treatment during the last five decades this lethal paediatric disease has been transformed into a chronic disorder with a median life expectancy of nowadays more than 50 years.

Current therapy is still mainly symptomatic, but meanwhile CFTR modulators have arrived to the clinic that target the basic defect in cystic fibrosis of impaired epithelial conductance for chloride and bicarbonate. There are two classes of CFTR modulators: Potentiators increase the activity of CFTR at the cell surface and correctors facilitate the translation, folding, maturation and trafficking of mutant CFTR to the cell surface and/or prevent its premature degradation. Already ten years ago the potentiator ivacaftor has been approved for the treatment of the small group of patients who carry a gating mutation in at least one of their two CFTR alleles. Ivacaftor is the first molecule that has been approved as a mutation-type specific medication for human use. Meanwhile the triple combination of the potentiator ivacaftor and the two correctors elexacaftor and tezacaftor is available for the treatment of the more than 90% of people with cystic fibrosis who harbour at least one CFTR allele that is responsive to this medication.

This monograph provides the reader with the background and on-going preclinical and clinical research for the development of mutation-type specific therapy of cystic fibrosis. Starting with the biology and biomarkers of CFTR in the context of cystic fibrosis, the reader gets insight into the basic and clinical research of CFTR modulators from bench to bedside. A large section of the book focuses on the clinical trials, post-approval observational studies and the real-world experience with the CFTR modulators.

When by the end of 2019 the spectacular clinical outcomes of the phase 3 studies on triple combination therapy were published, the NIH director Francis Collins, co-discoverer of the CFTR gene, commented this breakthrough in an editorial for the New England Journal of Medicine:

> "*Shortly after our identification of CFTR, I wrote a song entitled "Dare to Dream." The lyrics expressed hope that the gene discovery would lead to effective treatments for cystic fibrosis — that someday we would see "all our brothers and sisters breathing free." It is profoundly gratifying to see that this dream is coming true*" (Collins FS, NEJM 2019;381:1863-1865).

I cordially thank the many collaborators for their excellent timely contributions to this fast-moving and rewarding field, which has become a paradigm of personalized medicine.

Hannover, December 2021 *Burkhard Tümmler*

Authors

Editor

Burkhard Tümmler
Clinical Research Group „Molecular Pathology of Cystic Fibrosis"
Department for Paediatric Pneumology, Allergology and Neonatology
Hannover Medical School
Carl-Neuberg-Strasse 1
30625 Hannover, Germany

and

Biomedical Research in Endstage and Obstructive Lung Disease Hannover (BREATH),
Member of the German Center for Lung Research
Hanover Medical School
Hannover

Chapters 1.1., 1.6., 2.2., 3.2., 5.1., 5.3., 5.4.

Co-authors

Majid K.A. Al Salmani
Natural and Medical Sciences Research Center
University of Nizwa
P.O. Box 33
Postal Code 616, Nizwa, Sultanate of Oman

Chapter 1.3.

Jeffrey M. Beekman
Department of Pediatric Pulmonology
University Medical Center Utrecht
Wilhelmina Children's Hospital
Lundlaan 6
3584 EA, Utrecht, The Netherlands

Chapter 2.4.

Peter Braubach
Institute for Pathology
Hannover Medical School
Carl-Neuberg-Strasse 1
30625 Hannover
Germany

and

Biomedical Research in Endstage and Obstructive Lung Disease Hannover (BREATH), Member of the German Center for Lung Research
Hanover Medical School
Hannover

Chapter 2.5.

Jeng-Haur Chen
College of Chemistry and Life Sciences
Zhejiang Normal University
688 Yingbin Rd, Jinhua
Zhejiang Province, 321004 China

Chapter 1.4.

Jue Chen
Laboratory of Membrane Biophysics and Biology
The Rockefeller University
New York, NY, USA 10065

Chapter 1.2.

John P Clancy, MD
Cincinnati Children's Hospital Medical Center, MLC 2021
3333 Burnet Avenue
Cincinnati, OH, USA 45229

Chapter 1.1.

Anna-Maria Dittrich
Department for Paediatric Pneumology, Allergology and Neonatology
Hannover Medical School
Carl-Neuberg-Strasse 1
30625 Hannover
Germany

and

Biomedical Research in Endstage and Obstructive Lung Disease Hannover (BREATH), Member of the German Center for Lung Research
Hanover Medical School
Hannover

Chapter 2.5.

Sabina Gallati
Department of Genomic Medicine
Hirslanden Precise AG
Forchstrasse 452
CH-8702 Zollikon, Switzerland

Chapter 1.5.

Tanja Gonska
Department of Pediatrics
University of Toronto
Toronto, Canada

and

Physiology and Experimental Medicine
Research Institute and the Department of Pediatrics
Division of Gastroenterology, Hepatology and Nutrition
Hospital for Sick Children
Toronto

Chapter 2.1.

Simon Y. Gräber
Department of Pediatric Respiratory Medicine, Immunology and Critical Care Medicine
Charité – Universitätsmedizin Berlin
Augustenburger Platz 1
13353 Berlin, Germany

Chapter 2.3.

Bethan R. Hawley
School of Physiology, Pharmacology and Neuroscience
Biomedical Sciences Building
University of Bristol
University Walk
Bristol BS8 1TD, UK

Chapter 1.3.

Martin J. Hug
Pharmacy
Freiburg University Medical Center
Hugstetter St. 55
79106 Freiburg, Germany

Chapter 5.2.

Michal Irony-Tur Sinai
Department of Genetics
The Life Sciences Institute
Edmond J. Safra Campus
The Hebrew University
Jerusalem, Israel 91904

Chapter 4.

Danny Jonigk
Institute for Pathology
Hannover Medical School
Carl-Neuberg-Strasse 1
30625 Hannover
Germany

and

Biomedical Research in Endstage and Obstructive Lung Disease Hannover (BREATH), Member of the German Center for Lung Research
Hanover Medical School
Hannover

Chapter 2.5.

Till Frederik Kaireit
Institute for Diagnostic and Interventional Radiology
Hannover Medical School
Carl-Neuberg-Strasse 1
30625 Hannover
Germany

Chapter 3.2.

Batsheva Kerem
Department of Genetics
The Life Sciences Institute
Edmond J. Safra Campus
The Hebrew University
Jerusalem, Israel 91904

Chapter 4.

Eitan Kerem
Department of Pediatric Pulmonology and CF Center
Hadassah Medical Center and Faculty of Medicine
Hebrew University of Jerusalem
Jerusalem, Israel 91904

Chapter 4.

Jochen G. Mainz
Brandenburg Medical School (MHB), University
Cystic Fibrosis Center
Klinikum Westbrandenburg
Brandenburg an der Havel, Germany

Chapter 3.3.

Marcus A. Mall
Department of Pediatric Respiratory Medicine, Immunology and Critical Care Medicine
Charité – Universitätsmedizin Berlin
Augustenburger Platz 1
13353 Berlin, Germany

and

Berlin Institute of Health at Charité – Universitätsmedizin Berlin;
and German Center for Lung Research (DZL), associated partner site, Berlin, Germany

Chapter 2.3.

Yifat S. Oren
Department of Genetics
The Life Sciences Institute
Edmond J. Safra Campus
The Hebrew University
Jerusalem, Israel 91904

Chapter 4.

Sophia Theres Pallenberg
Department for Paediatric Pneumology, Allergology and Neonatology
Hannover Medical School
Carl-Neuberg-Strasse 1
30625 Hannover
Germanys

Chapter 2.2.

Isabelle Sermet-Gaudelus
Centre de Référence, Mucoviscidose et maladies apparentées. Site constitutif
Paris, France

and

INSERM U1121
Institut Necker Enfants Malades
Paris, France

Chapter 6.

David N. Sheppard
School of Physiology, Pharmacology and Neuroscience
Biomedical Sciences Building
University of Bristol
University Walk
Bristol BS8 1TD, UK

Chapter 1.3.

Mirjam Stahl
Department of Pediatric Respiratory Medicine, Immunology and Critical Care Medicine
Charité – Universitätsmedizin Berlin
Augustenburger Platz 1
13353 Berlin, Germany

Chapter 3.1.

Frauke Stanke
Clinical Research Group „Molecular Pathology of Cystic Fibrosis“
Department for Paediatric Pneumology, Allergology and Neonatology
Hannover Medical School
Carl-Neuberg-Strasse 1
30625 Hannover
Germany

and

Biomedical Research in Endstage and Obstructive Lung Disease Hannover (BREATH), Member of the German Center for Lung Research
Hanover Medical School
Hannover

Chapter 2.5.

Jens Vogel-Claussen
Institute for Diagnostic and Interventional Radiology
Hannover Medical School
Carl-Neuberg-Strasse 1
30625 Hannover
Germany

and

Biomedical Research in Endstage and Obstructive Lung Disease Hannover (BREATH), Member of the German Center for Lung Research
Hanover Medical School
Hannover

Chapter 3.2.

Min Wu
College of Chemistry and Life Sciences
Zhejiang Normal University
688 Yingbin Rd, Jinhua
Zhejiang Province, 321004 China

Chapter 1.4.

Contents

1. CFTR and cystic fibrosis

1.1. To set the stage: Cystic Fibrosis – etiology and significance

John P. Clancy and Burkhard Tümmler

Cystic fibrosis (CF) is a life-shortening, debilitating, and autosomal recessive disease affecting more than 80,000 people worldwide (Bell et al., 2020; Shteinberg et al., 2021). CF is caused by mutations in the gene that encodes the CF transmembrane conductance regulator protein (CFTR; Kerem et al., 1989; ☞ Chapter 1.5). This complex protein is an ABC transporter, distinguished by ATP binding and hydrolysis at nucleotide binding domains NBD-1 and NBD-2 to gate the chloride channel (Riordan et al., 1989; Riordan, 2008; ☞ Chapters 1.2. and 1.3.). CFTR is a chloride and bicarbonate channel (Anderson et al., 1991; Linsdell et al., 1997; Tang et al., 2009) that also regulates additional ion transporters, including other chloride channels, thiocyanate and glutathione transport, and the epithelial sodium channel (ENaC; Schwiebert et al., 1999; Stutts et al., 1995). In addition, CFTR is regulated by cAMP and PKA-dependent phosphorylation of its unique regulatory (R) domain (Cheng et al., 1991). CFTR is responsible for ion and fluid transport across the epithelia where it is expressed, along with serving an important role in airway host defense. Pulmonary CFTR expression is greatest in ionocytes that reside in small numbers in the lung and are specialized in ion transport (Montoro et al., 2018; Plasschaert et al., 2018), followed by submucosal glands and the pseudostratified epithelium of the medium and large airways and distal small-airway epithelial cells (Engelhardt et al., 1992; Engelhardt et al., 1994; Kälin et al., 1999; Shah et al., 2021).

> Although CFTR can be found in numerous tissues, its expression in the airways, the small and large intestines, pancreatic ducts, bile ducts, vas deferens, and sweat glands all have been connected directly to disease pathology. The universal feature of CF organ damage caused by CFTR deficiency is the buildup of mucus that is thick, tenacious, and dehydrated (Gustafsson et al., 2012).

It is hypothesized that the pathophysiology of CF airway disease is related directly to CFTR regulation of ion transport in surface-airway epithelia and submucosal glands, thus determining airway-surface liquid volume and mucus hydration (Stoltz et al., 2015). Without functional or quantitatively sufficient CFTR, cAMP-dependent chloride and bicarbonate transport is decreased resulting in net luminal dehydration and a reduced pH, which compromises normal bacterial killing by the innate immune system (Pezzulo et al., 2012). Mucus clearance is impaired (Gustafsson et al., 2012), which commences a chain of pathogenic steps including mucus stasis, airway obstruction, infection and inflammation (Shteinberg et al., 2021). CFTR deficiency in the airways yields exaggerated inflammation, with disproportionate release of pro-inflammatory cytokines that stimulate neutrophil-dominated inflammation (Konstan and Berger, 1997; Sagel et al., 2007). Over time, chronic airway colonization with bacterial pathogens, namely *Staphylococcus aureus* and *Pseudomonas aeruginosa* (Blanchard and Waters, 2019; Khanolkar et al., 2020), sustain a vicious cycle of infection, inflammation and remodeling that leads to airway structural damage, bronchiectasis, respiratory failure, and ultimately death in adulthood (Keown et al., 2020; Shteinberg et al., 2021).

Conventional treatment of CF has been mainly supportive, targeting downstream clinical manifestations that result from the loss of CFTR activity. These treatments are relatively effective to improve morbidity and survival, but result in a high care burden for CF patients and subsequent issues pertaining to adherence and quality of life (Bell et al., 2020). As we describe in this monograph, addressing the underlying cause of CF (i.e., restoring function to dysfunctional CFTR) offers the potential to dramatically change the disease course and to improve the quality of life of patients.

1.2. The Molecular Structures of CFTR

Jue Chen

The protein underlying cystic fibrosis is an ion channel named the cystic fibrosis transmembrane conductance regulator (CFTR). It belongs to the large family of ATP-binding cassette (ABC) transporters but functions as an anion channel (Anderson et al., 1991). Whereas other ABC transporters transport substrates thermodynamically uphill, CFTR conducts anions down their electrochemical gradients. In this chapter, we will describe the structures of CFTR determined by electron cryo-microscopy (cryo-EM) in two different conformations:

- the dephosphorylated, ATP-free form from zebrafish (Zhang and Chen, 2016) and man (Liu et al., 2017) and
- the phosphorylated, ATP-bound form from zebrafish (Zhang et al., 2017) and man (Zhang et al., 2018).

We will also discuss the structural features of CFTR that enable a mechanistic understanding of why this particular ABC transporter functions as an ion channel, how the channel activity is regulated, and how the drug ivacaftor interacts and potentiates CFTR (Liu et al., 2019).

1.2.1. CFTR is an unusual ABC transporter and an unusual ion channel

CFTR is a single polypeptide consisting of two homologous halves; each half contains a transmembrane domain (TMD) of six helices followed by a cytoplasmic nucleotide-binding domain (NBD; ☞ Figure 1.1A). The two TMDs form the anion conduction pathway and two NBDs bind and hydrolyze ATP. In addition, CFTR contains a regula-

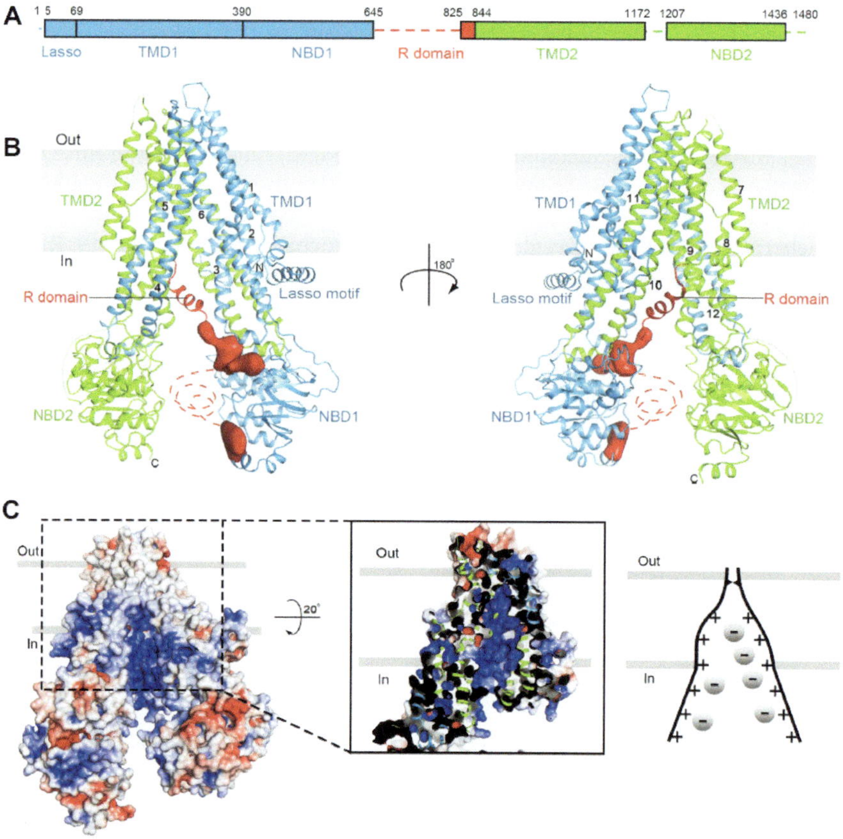

Figure 1.1: **Cryo-EM structure of human CFTR in the dephosphorylated, ATP-free conformation. A**: Schematic diagram showing the domain structure of CFTR. The numbers represent the range of residues visible in the cryo-EM map. **B**: Ribbon diagram of the overall structure. The EM densities shown in red correspond to unstructured region within the R domain. Regions not resolved in the structure are shown as dash lines. **C**: The electrostatic property of the interior surface of the pore and a schematic drawing of the funnel-shaped ion permeation pathway. Scale: red = negative (-5 kT/e), blue = positive (+5 kT/e).

tory (R) domain that plays an essential role in regulating the channel activity.

Unlike other ligand-gated ion channels, CFTR is not regulated by changes in the concentration of its ligand. Both phosphorylation of the R domain and ATP binding to the NBDs are required to open the CFTR channel (Cheng et al., 1991). As the intracellular concentration of ATP is near saturation and relatively constant, the activity of CFTR is predominantly regulated by cyclic AMP/protein kinase A (PKA)-dependent phosphorylation. Furthermore, CFTR consumes the ligand by catalyzing ATP hydrolysis. Similar to other ABC transporters, it contains two ATPase sites located at the interface of a closed NBD dimer. In CFTR, only one ATPase site is catalytically competent. The other site, which contains non-consensus residues including the Walker A motif of NBD1 and the ABC signature motif of NBD2, binds but does not hydrolyze ATP.

1.2.2. Structure of the non-phosphorylated CFTR

Incisive electrophysiology measurements have established that the open probability of CFTR is extremely low in the absence of phosphorylation and ATP. In this state, the molecular structure of CFTR resembles a typical ABC transporter in so-called "inward-facing" conformation with an inverted "V" shape (☞ Figure 1.1B). The 12 transmembrane helices segregate into two bundles that pack tightly in the membrane outer leaflet and progressively separate from the inner leaflet to the cytoplasm. The two TMDs are domain-swapped such that TM helices 1, 2, 3, and 6 pack against TM 10-11 to form one bundle; and TM 4 and 5 interact with TM 7, 8, 9, and 12 in TMD2 to form another bundle. The two NBDs, each attached to a TM helical bundle, are well-separated. The R domain, mostly unstructured, inserts between the cytoplasmic extension of the TMDs and the two NBDs.

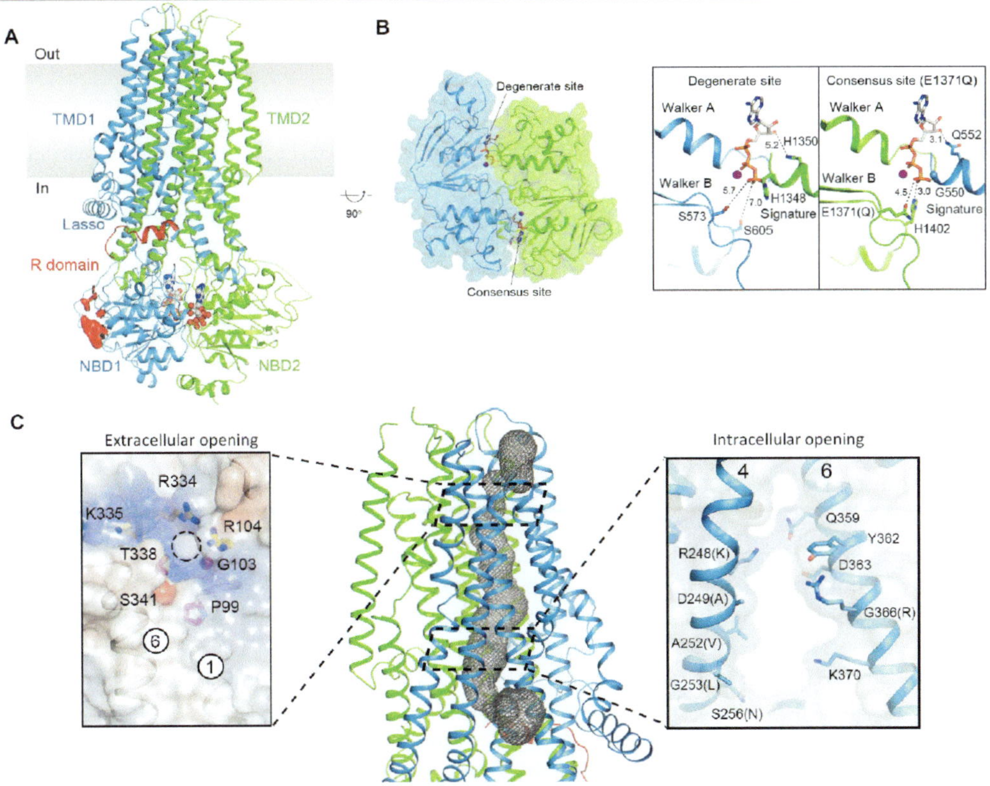

Figure 1.2: **Cryo-EM structure of human CFTR (E1371Q) in the phosphorylated, ATP-bound conformation.** **A**: Ribbon diagram. **B**: The closed NBD dimer. ATP is shown in ball-and-stick and distances are shown in Å. **C**: The ion translocation pathway. The gray mesh represents the pore, defined based on the size of a chloride ion (>1.7 Å radius). Residues lining the extracellular and intracellular openings are shown with side chains in the zoom-in views.

The ion conduction pathway, which is shaped like a funnel, lies at the interface of the two TMDs with a large cytosolic vestibule leading to a narrow transmembrane tunnel (☞ Figure 1.1C). The pore opens to the cytosol on one side of the molecule, between TM 4 and 6. A single gate near the extracellular surface closes the channel. The electrostatic surface of the ion conduction pathway is highly positive and lined with polar and charged residues, many of which have been functionally characterized to interact with anions including K95, Q98, E267, R303, S341, R352, and K1060. CFTR is a relatively non-selective anion channel, conducting many monovalent anions including thiocyanate, nitrate, bromide, chloride, iodide, fluoride, formate, and bicarbonate. Based on the structure, it seems likely that the selection of anions over cations in CFTR is largely attributed to the overall positive charge of pore rather than any individual residues.

1.2.3. Structure of phosphorylated CFTR in complex with ATP

Opening the CFTR pore requires phosphorylation of the R domain and binding of ATP to both NBDs. The structure of phosphorylated, ATP-bound CFTR, determined from a hydrolytic deficient mutant, is clearly different from that of the dephosphorylated, ATP-free CFTR (☞ Figure 1.2). Instead of an inverted "V", the molecule has an elongated shape (☞ Figure 1.2A). The two TM bundles pack tightly together to shield the ion-conduction pathway from the lipid bilayer. The two NBDs form a closed dimer, occluding two ATP molecules at their interface (☞ Figure 1.2B). The phosphorylated R domain, which remains largely unstructured, lies on the peripheral surface of the NBD dimer.

In this conformation, the ion conduction pathway is connected to both sides of the membrane: to the cytosol through the lateral opening TM 4 and 6 and to extracellular space through a small opening between TM 1 and TM 6 (☞ Figure 1.2C). The radius of the extracellular opening is about 1.2 Å, which would require further dilation to permeate ion or water molecules. Among the residues surrounding the extracellular opening, S341 and T338 have been proposed to gate the pore. Three positively charged residues, R104, R334, and K335, were also shown to influence anion conduction. Local conformational changes at this opening will result in a fully conductive channel.

The intracellular opening of the pore in the NBD-dimerized conformation is a unique feature of CFTR. Other ABC transporters that pump substrates thermodynamically uphill function via the alternating access mechanism, in which the translocation pathway opens only to one side of the membrane at a time. The intracellular gate in a typical ABC transporter is formed by a bundle of TM helices that pack closely in the NBD-dimerized conformation. In CFTR, this helical bundle is cracked open between TM helices 4 and 6 (☞ Figure 1.2C). Consequently, the ion conduction pathway is connected to the cytosol through this opening. CFTR has been described as a "broken" transporter since it permits ions flowing across the membrane bilayer. It is the cracked intracellular gate in the NBD-dimerized conformation that renders CFTR an ion channel instead of an active transporter.

1.2.4. Conformational changes leading to channel opening

Comparison of two CFTR structures identifies conformational changes necessary for channel opening (☞ Figure 1.3A). Upon phosphorylation and ATP binding, the NBDs move towards each other to form a closed dimer. The TMDs rotate essentially as rigid bodies in concert with the NBDs (☞ Figure 1.3B). In addition, conformational changes of the R domain and the TM helices reveal important aspects critical for CFTR gating.

It has been established that phosphorylation of the R domain increases the open probability of the CFTR channel and stimulates ATP hydrolysis. When de-phosphorylated, the R domain is wedged between TM helices 9, 10, and 12 and extends into the cytosol between the two NBDs. In this position, the unphosphorylated R domain functions as an auto-inhibitor, preventing NBD dimerization and channel opening (☞ Figure 1.3A). In the phosphorylated, ATP-bound conformation, the intracellular cleft in between the two halves of CFTR is completely closed off. The R domain packs along the outside surface of NBD1, away from the dimer interface. Disengagement of the R domain permits NBD dimerization, a conformational change necessary for channel opening and ATP hydrolysis (☞ Figure 1.3A).

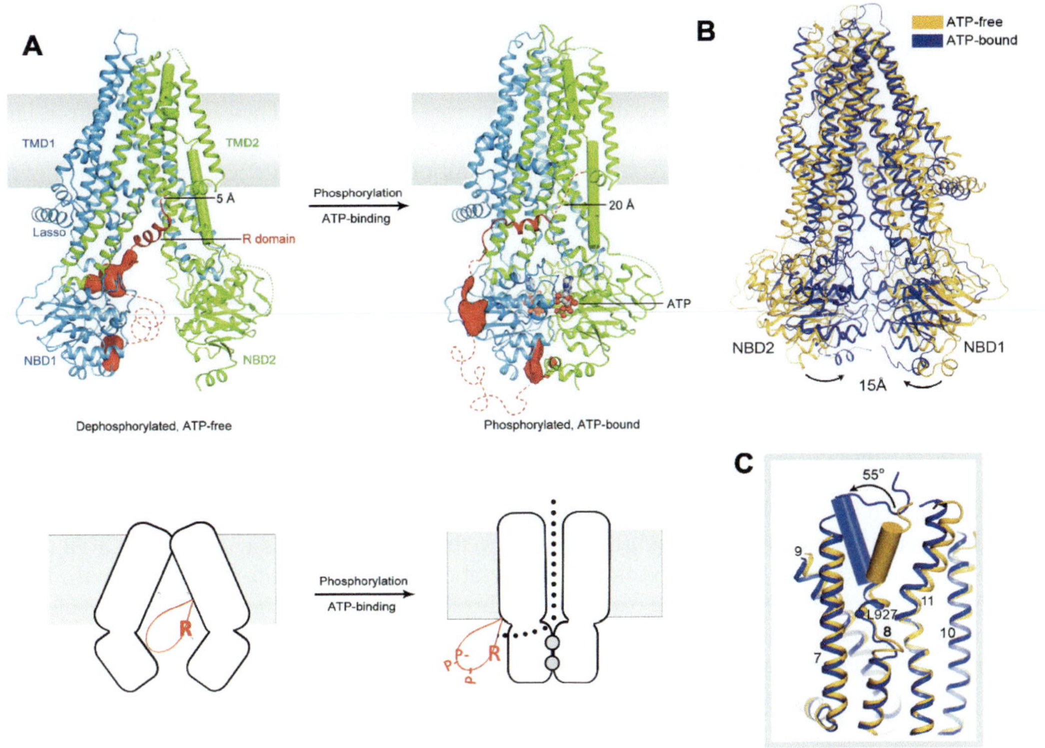

Figure 1.3: **Conformational changes upon phosphorylation and ATP-binding**. **A**: The overall structures. **B**: Superposition of the two structures, together with a zoom-in view. The outer leaflet segment of TM8 is shown in cylinder.

The R domain contains 19 predicted sites for protein kinase A (PKA); up to six have been found phosphorylated *in vivo*. Phosphorylation of multiple sites increases the overall negative change of the R domain. Such change could potentially lower its affinity at the intracellular space between the separated NBDs, thus facilitating R domain release from its inhibitory position. Alternatively, phosphorylation may promote interactions with the peripheral surface of NBD1, stabilizing the R domain away from the NBD dimer interface. In fact, the functional effects of phosphorylation can be imitated by simply deleting the R domain. Co-expression of the two halves of CFTR without the R domain results in an ATP-gated channel that opens independent of phosphorylation.

Another notable feature of CFTR is the discontinuity of helix TM8, which makes two sharp breaks inside the membrane creating a flexible hinge to facilitate gating (☞ Figure 1.3A, cylinder). The helical breaks free main-chain atoms from their secondary structure hydrogen bonds, thus rendering them available to interact with ions and water along the ion conduction pathway. Another potential functional consequence of breaks in helical secondary structure is that they can create flexible hinges to facilitate gating. Consistent with the latter hypothesis, the conformational changes elicited by phosphorylation and ATP binding involve a local conformational change around the helical break in TM8. Superimposed onto the global rigid body movement of the TMDs, the extracellular segments of TM8 and TM12 rotate approximately 50 degrees relative to the neighboring helices (☞ Figure 1.3B). A mutation in the TM8 loop, L927P, causes gating defects leading to cystic fibrosis, underscoring the functional importance of this hinge.

1.2.5. The TM hinge as a hotspot for CFTR potentiation

In recent years, small-molecule CFTR modulators have been developed, including correctors that increase the abundance of CFTR at the cell surface and potentiators that increase the ion flux of mutant CFTR. Currently, three correctors (elexacaftor, lumacaftor and tezacaftor) and one potentiator (ivacaftor) are available to patients. In addition, many other candidates are in the drug discovery pipeline (☞ Chapter 5.).

The cryo-EM structure of human CFTR in complex with ivacaftor shows that the potentiator binds CFTR inside the lipid bilayer, docking into a cleft at the protein-lipid interface (☞ Figure 1.4). In contrast to classic orthosteric sites of membrane bound receptors, the potentiator-binding site in CFTR is rather shallow. Approximately 40% of the molecular surface of ivacaftor is buried against CFTR; the remaining 60% is exposed to the hydrophobic region of the membrane. Mutagenesis studies identified four residues most important in drug recognition — their alanine substitutions nearly abolishing ivacaftor binding. Among them, S308 and F312 directly coordinate the oxoquinoline moiety through a hydrogen bond and a π-π stacking interaction, respectively (☞ Figure 1.4B). The other two residues, R933 and Y304A, hydrogen bond to main chain amides in the TM 8 hinge, thus stabilizing the overall structure of the binding site (☞ Figure 1.4B). These mutational effects indicate that hydrogen bonds are critical for ligand recognition in the low dielectric environment of the membrane.

Cryo-EM studies showed that another potentiator, GLPG1837, also binds CFTR at the same pocket as ivacaftor. Although the chemical structure of GLPG1837 differs from that of ivacaftor, residues interacting with GLPG1837 largely overlap with those engaging ivacaftor. Furthermore, replacing Y304 or S308 with an alanine increased the half maximal effective concentration values of GLPG1837 by 57- and 34-fold, respectively. The fact that two chemically distinct potentiators bind to the same site reveals a hotspot for CFTR potentiation. This binding site coincides with the helical break in TM8, suggesting that both molecules activate CFTR by stabilizing TM8 in its channel-opening configuration.

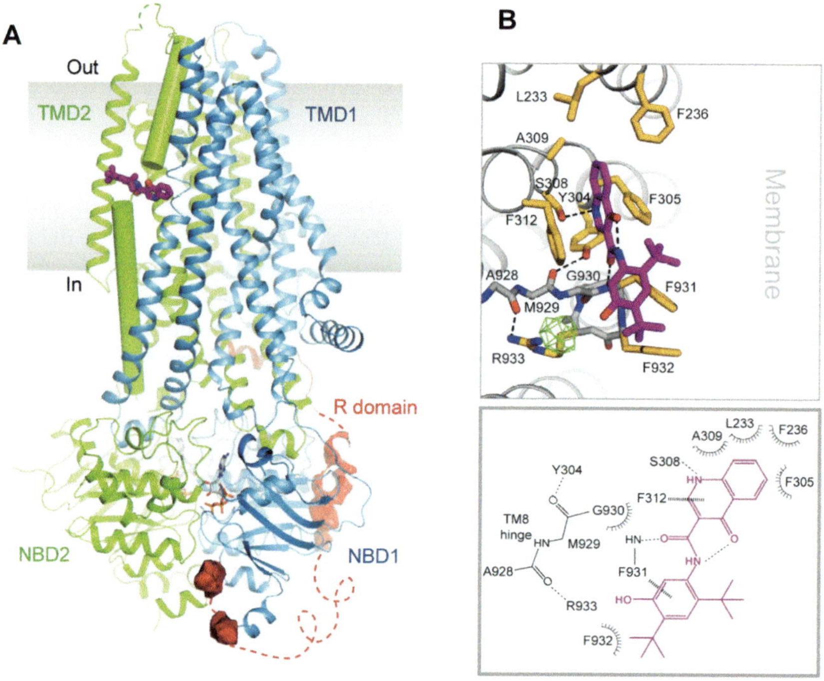

Figure 1.4: **Ivacaftor binds CFTR at the transmembrane hinge. A**: Overall structure of the phosphorylated, ATP-bound human CFTR in complex with ivacaftor (shown in magenta). TM8 is highlighted in cylinder representation. **B**: Zoom-in view of the ivacaftor-binding site. *Upper panel*: Residues within van der Waals distances are shown in yellow, and hydrogen bonds are depicted as dashed lines. An unknown density between R933 and ivacaftor is shown as green mesh. *Lower panel*: Schematic representations: black dashed lines = hydrogen bonds, blue vertical lines = aromatic interactions, spokes = hydrophobic interactions.

Summary

In this chapter, we described the structures of CFTR in both the dephosphorylated, channel-closed conformation and the phosphorylated, ATP-bound conformation (Zhang and Chen, 2016; Liu et al., 2017; Zhang et al., 2017; 2018). Comparing the two structures illustrates large conformational changes essential to CFTR channel gating. Finally, we discussed the finding of a hotspot for the action of CFTR potentiators ivacaftor and GLPG1837 (Liu et al., 2019).

1.3. Features of CFTR: an epithelial anion channel with complex regulation

Bethan R. Hawley, David N. Sheppard and Majid K.A. Al Salmani

The cystic fibrosis transmembrane conductance regulator (CFTR) is a low conductance anion-selective ion channel with complex regulation (Riordan et al., 1989; Hwang et al., 2018; Csanády et al., 2019). Its major role is to regulate chloride (Cl^-) and bicarbonate (HCO_3^-) ion movements across mucus covered epithelial tissues throughout the body (Saint-Criq and Gray, 2017). Three factors determine the function of CFTR: (i) the number of channels at the plasma membrane, (ii) the amount of time individual channels spend in the open, anion-conducting state and (iii) the ease of anion flow through open channels. Disturbances of any one of these factors occasionally singly, but typically in combination, cause CFTR dysfunction leading to the genetic disease cystic fibrosis (CF; Veit et al., 2016). Here, we review briefly the relationship between CFTR structure and function. This knowledge is critical to understand how pathogenic variants in the *CFTR* gene cause disease and the mechanisms of action of CFTR modulators that restore function to faulty channels.

1.3.1. The functional architecture of CFTR

Based on its amino acid sequence and domain organisation, CFTR is an ATP-binding cassette (ABC) transporter (Hwang et al., 2018; Csanády et al., 2019). However, its ion channel function sets CFTR apart from all other ABC transporters, most of whom pump diverse substrates across cell membranes (Holland et al., 2003). CFTR is assembled from 1,480 amino acids organised into five major domains:

- two membrane-spanning domains (MSDs),
- two nucleotide-binding domains (NBDs) and
- a regulatory domain (RD)

arranged in two MSD-NBD motifs separated by the RD (Riordan et al., 1989). The MSDs are composed of six transmembrane segments, which assemble to form a gated pore for transmembrane anion flow. Phosphorylation of the RD by protein kinase A is a prerequisite for CFTR activity. Thereafter, anion flow through the CFTR pore is tightly controlled by cycles of ATP binding and hydrolysis at the NBDs. Conformational changes initiated by ATP binding at the NBDs are communicated to the MSDs by the intracellular loops (ICLs; Mornon et al., 2008; Serohijos et al., 2008). Upon opening of the channel gate, anions flow passively through the CFTR pore down a favourable electrochemical gradient. Therefore, even though each CFTR domain is a separate functional unit, CFTR activity is dependent on dynamic structural interactions between individual domains.

1.3.2. Phosphorylation-dependent regulation of CFTR: the RD

PKA-dependent phosphorylation initiates CFTR activity by targeting the RD (Hwang et al., 2018; Csanády et al., 2019), the first unique feature of CFTR identified; others have emerged particularly through structural studies. The RD is distinguished by multiple consensus phosphorylation sites for PKA (Riordan et al., 1989), many charged amino acid residues (Riordan et al., 1989) and no stable secondary or tertiary structure (e.g. Zhang et al., 2018). Among the multiple phosphorylation sites, which decorate the RD, those at serine S660, S700, S737, S795 and S813 are the most important for CFTR regulation by PKA. These sites were phosphorylated *in vivo* by cAMP agonists (Cheng et al., 1991), while the largest reduction of CFTR activity was achieved with the simultaneous mutation of S660, S737, S795 and S813 (Chang et al., 1993; Rich et al., 1993). These and other data (e.g. Hegedüs et al., 2009), argue that PKA stimulation of CFTR is redundant with no one individual phosphoserine essential for CFTR function. The data also suggest that there are context-dependent functional interactions between different phosphoserines to precisely control CFTR-mediated anion transport.

The RD was initially proposed to regulate CFTR by keeping the channel closed when dephosphorylated (Rich et al., 1991). Supporting this idea, structural studies demonstrated that the unphosphorylated RD is positioned between the two MSD-NBD motifs, interacting with NBD1, MSD2, NBD2 and the C-terminus (e.g. Liu et al., 2017). Upon RD phosphorylation, addition of negative charge to the RD or deletion of a large part of the domain, channel inhibition is relieved (Rich et al., 1991; Chang et al., 1993; Rich et al., 1993). Structural studies have revealed that PKA-dependent phosphorylation leads to RD disengagement from between the NBDs and binding to the lasso motif, allowing regulation of CFTR channel gating by ATP-driven NBD dimerization (e.g. Zhang et al., 2018). Importantly, the activity of phosphorylated wild-type CFTR exceeded greatly that of variants, which did not require phosphorylation to open in the presence of ATP (Chang et al., 1993; Rich et al., 1993). These data suggested that the phosphorylated RD might stimulate CFTR activity. Consistent with this idea, PKA-dependent phosphorylation enhanced ATP binding and hydrolysis at the NBDs to accelerate the rate of channel opening (Li et al., 1996; Winter and Welsh, 1997; Liu et al., 2017). Thus, the RD does not simply function as an "on-off" switch, but as a dynamic integrator of CFTR function (Bozoky et al., 2013). Through interactions with the NBDs and MSDs at multiple sites and communication with CFTR-interacting proteins, the RD orchestrates CFTR activity (Guggino and Stanton, 2006; Bozoky et al., 2013).

1.3.3. Regulation of CFTR channel gating by ATP binding and hydrolysis: the NBDs

The gating pattern of the CFTR channel describes the frequency with which the protein transits be-

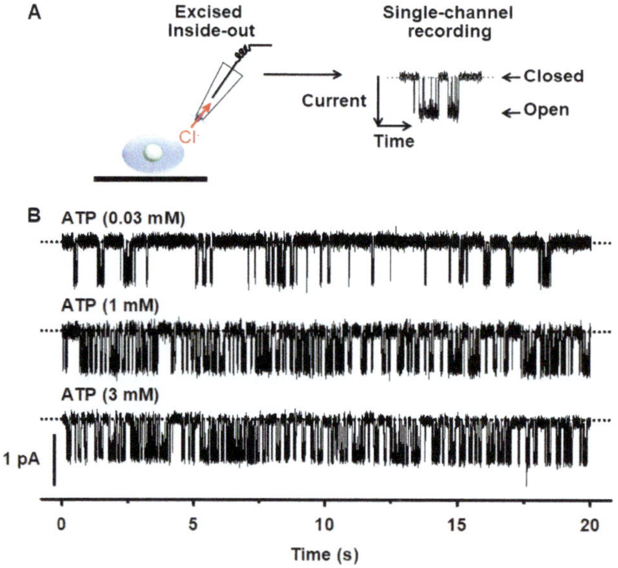

Figure 1.5: **CFTR channel gating is regulated by ATP. A**: Schematic representation of the excised inside-out configuration of the patch-clamp technique used to record current flow through CFTR. When the membrane patch contains a single CFTR Cl^- channel, conformation changes corresponding to channel opening and closing can be monitored in real time. Note that Cl^- flow from the bath (intracellular) to pipette (extracellular) solution corresponds to downward deflections of the current record. **B**: Representative recordings of a wild-type CFTR Cl^- channel in an excised inside-out membrane patch from a C127 cell heterologously expressing wild-type human CFTR. The recordings were made in the continuous presence of PKA (75 nM) and the indicated concentrations of ATP in the intracellular solution. To magnify channel openings, voltage was clamped at −50 mV and a large Cl^- concentration gradient imposed across the membrane patch (internal [Cl^-], 10 mM; external [Cl^-], 147 mM). Dotted lines indicate where the channel is closed and downward deflections of the recording correspond to channel openings. Modified with permission from Li and Sheppard (2009).

tween closed (non-conducting) and open (conducting) states. The gold standard method to evaluate CFTR channel activity is single-channel recording using the patch-clamp technique. This technique detects transitions of the channel between closed and open states in real time at the resolution of single molecules fluttering open and closed on a millisecond time-scale (☞ Figure 1.5A). Once CFTR is fully phosphorylated, increasing the ATP concentration on the intracellular side of the membrane enhances the frequency, but not the duration of channel openings (☞ Figure 1.5B). Unique to CFTR, channel closure depends on the enzymatic activity of the NBDs, which destroys the ligand ATP to make the CFTR gating cycle irreversible (Hwang et al., 2018; Csanády et al., 2019).

The NBDs of CFTR are composed of three subdomains: the F1-type ATP binding core, the ABC α and the ABC β, distinguished by conserved amino acid sequences (Lewis et al., 2004). In addition, NBD1 contains a 32 residue intrinsically disordered segment called the regulatory insertion (RI) not found in other ABC transporters (Lewis et al., 2004). For several reasons, the RI is of special interest. First, deletion of the RI rescues the expression and function of the predominant pathogenic CFTR variant F508del (Aleksandrov et al., 2010). Second, functional studies suggest that the RI regulates CFTR channel gating (Csanaìdy et al., 2005; Scholl et al., 2021). Third, structural studies demonstrate that NBD1 can adopt an alternative conformation, where the RI is partially folded (Scholl et al., 2021). Taken together, the data suggest that the RI might function as a conformational switch to regulate CFTR function.

The NBDs of CFTR function as a head-to-tail dimer with two ATP-binding sites located at the dimer interface assembled from sequences contributed by both NBDs. One site is formed by the Walker A and B motifs of NBD1 and the LSGGQ (or ABC signature) motif of NBD2 (termed ATP-binding site 1). The other site is formed by the Walker A and B motifs of NBD2 and the LSGGQ motif of NBD1 (termed ATP-binding site 2; Lewis et al., 2004; Zhang et al., 2018). Tight dimerization of the two NBDs, achieved by ATP occupancy of both its binding sites, is required for optimal ATPase activity and channel gating (Kidd et al., 2004; Vergani et al., 2005).

However, many studies demonstrated asymmetries in the structure and function of the NBDs (for review, ☞ Hwang et al., 2018; Csanády et al., 2019), arguing that the two ATP-binding sites are not equivalent in function. For example, using photoaffinity labelling, Aleksandrov et al. (2002) demonstrated that NBD1 (i.e. ATP-binding site 1) stably binds nucleotides, whereas NBD2 (i.e. ATP-binding site 2) rapidly hydrolyses them. Vergani et al. (2005) integrated the results of biochemical, functional and structural studies of the NBDs to propose the ATP-driven NBD dimerization model of CFTR channel gating. In this model, CFTR channel gating is controlled by ATP binding and hydrolysis at site 2 driving cycles of NBD dimer assembly and disassembly. Of note, the authors demonstrated that arginine(R)555 (NBD1) and threonine(T)1246 (NBD2) are energetically coupled in open, but not closed channels, arguing that the NBDs undergo dynamic reorganisation during channel gating (Vergani et al., 2005). During the gating cycle, site 1 remains tightly closed around a bound ATP molecule, whereas site 2 undergoes conformational changes, closing following ATP binding, but opening after ATP cleavage to release the products of ATP hydrolysis (Vergani et al., 2005; Tsai et al., 2010; Szollosi et al., 2011). Thus, the NBDs act as an engine to power dynamic structural rearrangements in the MSDs, which gate the channel pore with the rate of ATP binding and hydrolysis acting as a timing mechanism to control anion flow through CFTR.

1.3.4. Anion flow through the CFTR pore: the MSDs

The MSDs assemble to form a transmembrane pore, which mediates the passive flow of anions across the plasma membrane. Interestingly, the architecture of the CFTR pore is asymmetric in two ways:

- First, the two MSDs do not contribute equally. Transmembrane segment 6 (M6) in MSD1 plays the dominant role in specifying the pore properties of CFTR (Hwang et al., 2018). Residues along the length of M6 and M12 and in sections of M1, M3, M4, M5, M9, M10 and M11 line the pore (for review, ☞ Hwang et al., 2018).
- Second, the CFTR pore resembles an asymmetric hourglass with deep intracellular and shallow

extracellular vestibules separated by a constriction towards the external side of the pore (for review, ☞ Linsdell, 2017; ☞ Figure 1.6).

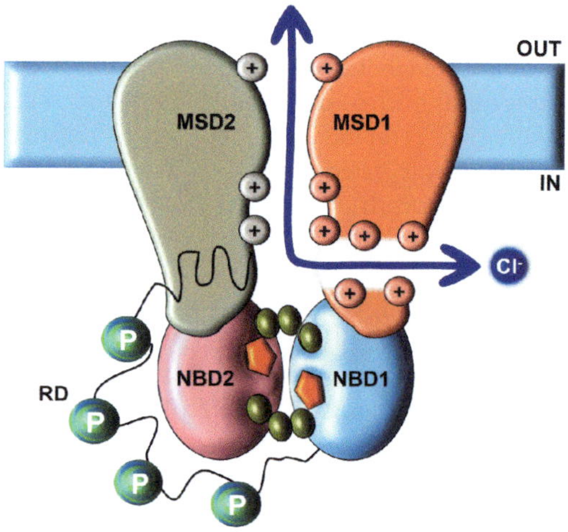

Figure 1.6: **Architecture of the CFTR pore.** Schematic representation of the CFTR pore based on structural and functional data. On the intracellular side of the membrane, anions enter the pore through a lateral tunnel within the ICLs beneath MSD1 connected to the intracellular vestibule, whereas they exit the pore on the extracellular side directly from the extracellular vestibule. The pore is lined by positively charged arginine and lysine residues, which stream anions through the channel. ATP is presented as three dark balls linked to a pentagon. Reproduced with permission from Al Salmani et al. (2020).

On the extracellular side of the channel, anions readily enter the extracellular vestibule and are funnelled toward the pore constriction (Zhang and Chen, 2016; Linsdell, 2017). By contrast, the intracellular vestibule is not directly accessible from the cytoplasm (Zhang and Chen, 2016; Linsdell, 2017; ☞ Figure 1.6). Instead, the vestibule is reached by a lateral tunnel within the ICLs beneath M4 and M6, which runs parallel to the plane of the plasma membrane (Hoffmann et al., 2018; Li et al., 2018; Zhang et al., 2018). At the tunnel's mouth and within the vestibules, positively charged residues maximise anion flow towards the pore constriction by electrostatic repulsion (Zhang and Chen, 2016; Linsdell, 2017; Hwang et al., 2018).

The pore constriction determines the anion selectivity of CFTR. This region, where the CFTR pore narrows to ~5.3 Å in diameter is located between leucine(L)102-isoleucine(I)106 (M1) and T338-S341 (M6; Linsdell and Hanrahan, 1998; Hwang et al., 2018). The permeation of anions through the CFTR pore follows a lyotropic sequence, determined by the hydration energy of anions with large, weakly hydrated anions being most permeant (Smith et al., 1999). Interestingly, the CFTR pore can switch between conformations permeable to Cl^- and HCO_3^-. When the intracellular $[Cl^-]$ falls below 10 mM, with-no-lysine kinase 1 (WNK1) dilates the CFTR pore by an unknown mechanism to enhance CFTR-mediated HCO_3^- permeation (Kim et al., 2020). This change in the anion selectivity of CFTR likely allows pancreatic duct cells to achieve the high rates of HCO_3^- secretion necessary to produce HCO_3^--rich pancreatic juice (Kim et al., 2020).

The pore constriction is the location of an ATP-controlled gate within the CFTR pore formed by residues towards the external end of M1, M6, M8 and M12 (Gao and Hwang, 2015; Zhang and Chen, 2016). Of note, M8 contains a unique discontinuous region, not found in other ABC transporters, which likely forms a flexible hinge that gates the CFTR pore (Zhang and Chen, 2016). The unusual structure of M8 together with the loss of a second gate located on the intracellular side of the MSDs are the evolutionary changes that transformed CFTR from an active transporter into an ion channel (Hwang et al., 2018).

1.3.5. Structural rearrangements of CFTR domains during channel gating

Comparison of the dephosphorylated ATP-free and phosphorylated ATP-bound structures of human CFTR provides an explanation for how ATP binding at the NBDs opens the channel pore formed by the MSDs (Liu et al., 2017; Zhang et al., 2018). In the dephosphorylated ATP-free state, the two MSD-NBD motifs form an inverted V shape with the MSDs locked together near the extracellular side of the membrane and the NBDs separated by the RD (Liu et al., 2017; ☞ Figure 1.7).

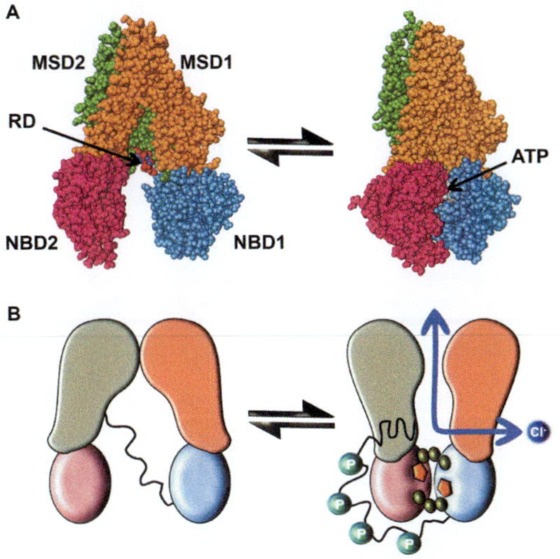

Figure 1.7: **Phosphorylation- and ATP-dependent reorganisation of CFTR domains. A**: The structures of human CFTR in the absence (left) and presence (right) of RD phosphorylation and ATP binding at the NBDs (PBD ids: 5UAK and 6MSM). **B**: Schematic representation of the two CFTR structures shown in A revealing the organisation of the different domains, the ATP-binding sites and the ATP-dependent gating movements. Reproduced with permission from Al Salmani et al. (2020).

On phosphorylation, the RD is displaced and ATP drives NBD dimerization, leading to conformation changes in the MSDs, which result in the two MSD-NBD motifs aligning vertically to each other (Vergani et al., 2005; Zhang et al., 2018; ☞ Figure 1.7). Molecular dynamics simulations suggest that M8 swings out to open the CFTR pore with its movement coordinated with that of M6, M7 and M12 (Hoffmann et al., 2018). The reorientation of the MSDs during the transition from the dephosphorylated ATP-free to phosphorylated ATP-bound structures packs transmembrane segments together to shield the CFTR pore from the lipid bilayer (Zhang et al., 2018). Consistent with functional data (Bai et al., 2011), this movement causes the intracellular vestibule to narrow. However, in the phosphorylated ATP-bound structure, the CFTR pore is too narrow in the region of the pore constriction for Cl^- to pass. It is therefore possible that a different structure might represent the open-channel configuration observed with the patch-clamp technique.

Summary

CFTR is a unique ABC transporter that functions as a low-conductance anion-selective channel gated by cycles of ATP binding and hydrolysis at its NBDs and regulated tightly by the RD, an intrinsically disordered protein segment distinguished by multiple consensus phosphorylation sites. By regulating the quantity and quality of epithelial secretions, CFTR plays a pivotal role in epithelial physiology, best illustrated by the consequences of its dysfunction in CF.

1.4. Basic defect in cystic fibrosis

Min Wu and Jeng-Haur Chen

Cystic fibrosis (CF) is an inherited genetic disease, caused by mutations in the gene encoding the cystic fibrosis transmembrane conductance regulator (CFTR), a Cl^- channel predominantly found in the apical membrane of epithelial cells (Shteinberg et al., 2021a). CF-associated mutations may cause structural defects in CFTR, leading to channel dysfunction and followed by a variety of epithelial disorders in the lung, liver, intestine, pancreas, sweat gland and reproductive ducts (Shteinberg et al., 2021a). Nowadays, progressive tissue damage caused by inflammation, mucus accumulation and bacterial infection in the lung is responsible for the majority of morbidity and mortality in CF (Stoltz et al., 2015).

CFTR transports Cl^- to control fluid absorption or secretion by epithelia (☞ Figure 1.8; Stoltz et al., 2015) while the channel also moderately conducts HCO_3^- to regulate intra- and extracellular pH (☞ Figure 1.8; Zajac et al., 2021). In addition, CFTR acts as an intracellular regulator that by protein-protein interactions forms macromolecular complexes with several intracellular regulatory proteins (☞ Figure 1.8; Zhang et al., 2017). Consequently, CFTR dysfunction in CF epithelia may cause defective transepithelial Cl^- and HCO_3^- transport and abnormal cellular function (☞ Figure 1.8; Shteinberg et al., 2021a; Stoltz et al., 2015; Zhang et al., 2017). Which one of above defects plays a major role in the pathogenesis of CF remains a major task in the field, since knowing the dominant defect of the disease allows us to find effective treatments for CF.

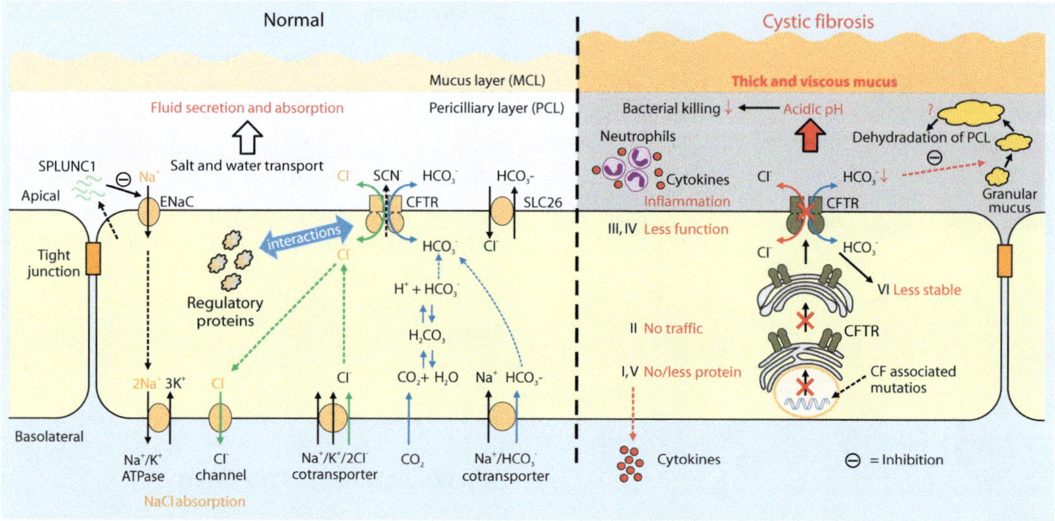

Figure 1.8: **Dysfunction of CFTR leads to CF defects in airway epithelia.** Left section shows CFTR-dependent Cl^- and HCO_3^- transport and interactions with regulatory proteins in epithelial cells. Other apical and basolateral transporters further contribute to CFTR-mediated transepithelial electrolyte transport, pH regulation and fluid secretion and absorption. Airway surface liquid (ASL) contains the mucus layer (MCL) and periciliary layer (PCL). Abbreviations: ENaC = epithelial Na^+ channel, SLC26 = solute carrier 26 proteins (Note, some SLC26 proteins may form Cl^- channels). Right section indicates 6 classes (I - VI) of CF-associated mutations affecting CFTR expression and function. Text and lines in red indicate defects that occur in CF epithelia (☞ text for more details).

1.4.1. CF mutations cause molecular defects in the CFTR Cl^- channel

Currently, more than 2,000 CF-associated mutations have been identified (Zhang et al., 2017). According to their actions impairing CFTR function, these mutations have been grouped into 6 classes (☞ Figure 1.9 and Chapter 1.6.). The most common CF mutation p.Phe508del, deleting a phenylalanine residue at position 508 and carried by about 90% patients with CF (Amaral and Farinha, 2013), causes significant defects in CFTR protein processing and channel gating (Cai et al., 2011), and weakened channel activation by cAMP stimulation (Ostedgaard et al., 2011) and gating stimulation by acidic intracellular pH (Chen et al., 2017). The functional loss of p.Phe508del-CFTR may be

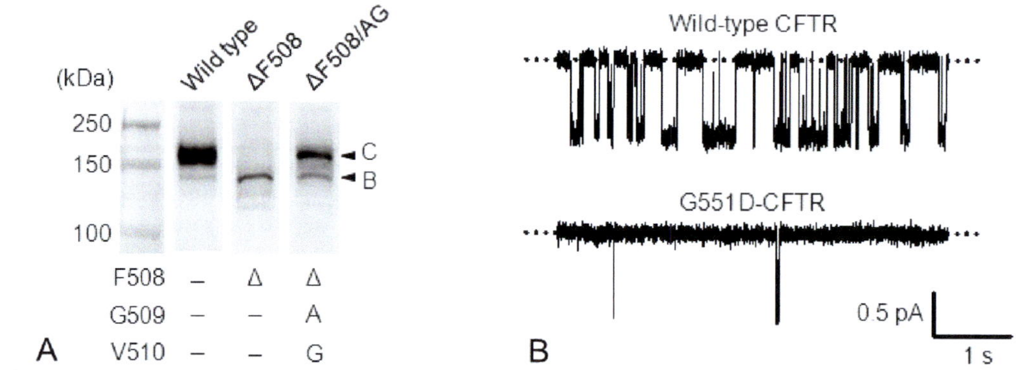

Figure 1.9: **CF-associated mutations impair CFTR processing and channel gating. A**: Effects of the ΔF508 mutation on CFTR maturation. Arrows indicate positions of CFTR with Band B (B, core glycosylated protein) or Band C (C, fully glycosylated protein). The G509A/V510G (AG) mutations shift the G509 residue one position backward in the peptide and greatly rescue ΔF508-CFTR processing. **B**: Channel gating of wild-type and mutant G551D-CFTR at 1 mM ATP and 75 nM PKA. Single-channel traces of 5 seconds duration are shown. Dotted lines indicate the closed state of CFTR and downward deflections correspond to channel openings (☞ text for more details).

partly due to minor structural alterations by the position shift of the Gly509 residue (☞ Figure 1.9; Chen et al., 2019), misfolding of NBD1 (Farinha and Canato, 2017) and abnormal domain-domain interactions (Farinha and Canato, 2017). CFTR potentiators that improv channel activity, e.g., ivacaftor in combination with CFTR correctors that enhance protein expression, e.g., elexacaftor and tezacaftor, are transforming the care of patients with CF and the p.Phe508del mutation (Barry and Taylor-Cousar, 2021).

1.4.2. CF-associated mutations cause deficits of CFTR function

CFTR conducts both Cl^- and HCO_3^- across the apical membrane of epithelia with the permeation ratio of about 4 : 1 (Cl^- : HCO_3^-; Poulsen et al., 1994). The multiple ion selectivity of CFTR challenges the original hypothesis that loss of Cl^- transport in CF is chiefly responsible for pathogenesis of diseases (Sheppard et al., 1993) since HCO_3^- transport might be coincidently reduced in mutant CFTR. The lack of HCO_3^- transport is found associated with pancreatic insufficiency in patients with CF (Choi et al., 2001) and may lower luminal surface pH, attenuating bacterial killing (Pezzulo et al., 2012). Moreover, defects in both Cl^- and HCO_3^- transport of the submucosal gland is proposed to be responsible for abnormal mucus movement over airway epithelia of CF newborn pigs (Hoegger et al., 2014). Mucus is initially secreted in a granular form (☞ Figure 1.8) and then by absorbing periciliary liquid expands more than 1,000 fold of its original volume (Zajac et al., 2021). Thus, defective ion and water movement in CF may affect mucus expansion and movement over airway epithelia (Abdullah et al., 2017).

As a cellular regulator, CFTR through its N- and C-termini and regulatory domain interacts with a variety of intracellular proteins, such as Na^+/H^+ exchanger regulatory factor 2, Na^+/H^+ exchanger isoform 3, SLC26 Cl^-/HCO_3^- exchangers, and anti-sigma factor antagonist domain (Bozoky et al., 2013; Li and Naren, 2010; Zhang et al., 2017). Disruption of these interactions in CF may lead to cellular defects, which need the development of new treatments to restore normal function (Zhang et al., 2017). Moreover, airway epithelia secrete SPLUNC1 peptides into the periciliary fluid (☞ Figure 1.8), where the peptide binds the extracellular domain of the epithelial Na^+ channel (ENaC) leading to channel internalization (Webster and Tarran, 2018). Furthermore, stimulated by bacteria and other pathogens, CF epithelia and inflammatory cells release cytokines onto airway epithelia (☞ Figure 1.8) to elicit and enhance inflammation responses (Roesch et al., 2018). These findings may somehow contribute to the mechanisms of CF pathogenesis caused by CFTR dysfunction.

1.4.3. Functional deficits of CFTR mutants lead to defects in epithelial function

Epithelial disorders due to CFTR dysfunction impairs bacteria eradication by both epithelial innate defense and the mucociliary clearance mechanism (Shteinberg et al., 2021a; Stoltz et al., 2015), which may result in mucus accumulation and sustained inflammation, the hallmark of CF airway disease (Shteinberg et al., 2021a). It has been proposed that lack of CFTR expression may upregulate the ENaC activity, leading to Na^+ hyperabsorption that may dehydrate airway surface liquid (ASL) and impair mucus movement and bacteria eradication, leading to CF lung disease (Boucher, 2007). Although ASL depletion is observed in cultured airway epithelia (Matsui et al., 1998) and CF-like lung disease occurs in transgenic mice with overexpression of ENaC (Mall et al., 2004), ASL height is not different between wild-type and CF newborn pigs (Chen et al., 2010) and the inhibition of ENaC activity by CFTR is still in debate (Berdiev et al., 2009; Luan et al., 2021). Therefore, it is suggested that CF airway does not hyperabsorb Na^+ (for details ☞ the review Stoltz et al., 2015).

Lack of HCO_3^- secretion is also widely observed in CF epithelia of the liver bile duct, pancreas, intestine and reproductive ducts (Betapudi et al., 2021; Kunzelmann et al., 2017). Other defects in CF epithelia-lined organs include inflammation and microbiome changes in the gastrointestinal duct (Sathe et al., 2021), activation of the Rous sarcoma oncogene cellular homolog (Src) in cholangiocytes of the bile duct (Betapudi et al., 2021) and deficiencies in sex hormone and infertility in CF males (Shteinberg et al., 2021b).

Possibly caused by inflammation, malnutrition, organ dysfunction and insufficient hormone secretion, systemic CF defects can be found in many patients with CF, e.g., diabetes mellitus (Coderre et al., 2021) and IGF-1 deficiency (Lavi et al., 2020). Such deficits may intensively influence physiological function, weight and growth of the whole body and complicate symptoms and treatments for patients with CF (Coderre et al., 2021; Lavi et al., 2020). With various defects in multiple organs, CF is characterized as a multisystem disease (Shteinberg et al., 2021a).

1.4.4. CFTR dysfunction causes defects in non-epithelial tissues

CFTR has been found in non-epithelial cells, such as endothelial cells, cardiac myocytes, vascular smooth muscle cells, monocytes, macrophages and neurons (Poore et al., 2021; Reznikov, 2017; Roesch et al., 2018). Disruption of CFTR in these cells may alter cell and tissue properties and functions, resulting in systemic disorders such as cerebrovascular dysfunction (Poore et al., 2021) and ventilatory responses (Reznikov, 2017). However, further investigation is still required to confirm the correlation between CFTR dysfunction and the causes of these defects.

In summary, CF-associated mutations induce structural defects that disrupt CFTR production, channel activity and regulatory function (Shteinberg et al., 2021a). Lack of HCO_3^- transport due to low CFTR activity may acidify ASL, becoming an important cause of CF pathogenesis (Stoltz et al., 2015). This defect is not only seen universally among CF organs but also affects bacterial killing by airway epithelia and alters mucus properties among ductal organs (Kunzelmann et al., 2017; Stoltz et al., 2015). Although ASL pH in CF epithelia is consistently found to be more acidic than non-CF epithelia in cell culture (Kunzelmann et al., 2017; Zajac et al., 2021), data from *in vivo* measurements on human airway are controversial (Zajac et al., 2021). Several factors, such as low luminal partial CO_2 pressure and a variety of pH regulatory transporters present in epithelial cells (Zajac et al., 2021), may weaken the impact of HCO_3^- deficiency by mutant CFTR in CF airway. In addition, defective unfolding of MUC5B mucus in CF is also irrelevant to HCO_3^- and pH levels (Abdullah et al., 2017). Nevertheless, restoration of HCO_3^- transport in CF epithelia is an important goal for future treatments. Thus, dissecting in detail the individual contribution of multiple defects to CF pathogenesis may further elucidate the origins of the disease.

1.5. Population genetics of *CFTR* mutations

Sabina Gallati

CF causing mutations have existed for more than 50,000 years and many are strongly associated with specific populations. The most common *CFTR* mutation, the 3-bp deletion F508del (c.1521_1523delCTT; p.Phe508del according to the HGVS nomenclature) in exon 11 (legacy exon 10), accounts worldwide for approximately 60-70% of all CF chromosomes with considerably variable frequencies depending on populations and geographical locations (WHO report 2004, http://www.who.int/genomics/publications/en/). There is a clear North West to South East gradient in F508del frequency across Europe with a maximum of 100% in the isolated Faroe Islands of Denmark and a minimum of about 22% in Turkey. The Canadian and North American populations present with a F508del frequency of 68-71%, whereas Hispanic populations and American Blacks show frequencies between 42% and 48%. The overall frequency of non-F508del mutations is low, except for some population specific mutations such as e.g. W1282X accounting for around 48% of CF chromosomes in Ashkenazi Jews or 621+1G>T accounting for 23% of French Canadian CF chromosomes.

More than 2,100 *CFTR* variants have been reported so far to the Cystic Fibrosis Genetic Analysis Consortium (CFGAC; www.genet.sickkids.on.ca), of which almost 80% are classified as causing CF, 7.3% as unclear and 12.7% as benign. Besides the F508del, there are another 22 relatively common mutations causing classic CF and reported to occur at a frequency of 0.1% or higher by the American College of Medical Genetics (ACMG; Watson et al., 2004). Another 21 variants with a frequency of ≥0.1% as well as 144 variants with a frequency of ≥0.01% were functionally investigated within the framework of the CFTR2 project and found to be consistent with CF disease (www.cftr2.org; as of September 2021). A few mutations with an unusually high frequency in specific populations indicate founder effect genetic drift. The remaining mutations represent rare or even individual sequence changes that are distributed throughout the entire gene.

The identification of the *CFTR* gene in 1989 raised new hope for a causative treatment targeting the basic defect of CF. However, therapeutic approaches that would benefit all CF patients independent of their genotype such as *CFTR* gene addition or gene replacement, were not successful so far. In contrast, novel therapeutic tools have been developed focussing on the correction of specific *CFTR* mutations and highlighting the need for careful characterisation of each patient's genotype towards individualised medicine.

Mutations (missense, nonsense, frameshift, splice, small and large in-frame deletions and insertions) contribute to the phenotype by their nature and position in the gene and can be grouped into different classes based on known or predicted functional consequences for the protein (Lubamba et al., 2012, MacDonald et al., 2007, Welsh et al., 1993). Class I (mainly nonsense, frameshift, and splice site) and class II mutations (e.g. F508del) promote no functional CFTR at the apical membrane, whereas in classes III to V the protein is expressed on the cellular surface but with limited function such as defective regulation (III, e.g. G551D), reduced conductance (IV, e.g. R117H, R347H) or reduced splicing efficiency (V, e.g. 5T, 3849+10kbC>T). Class VI mutations (e.g. Q1412X, 4279insA) lead to a marked instability of an otherwise fully processed und functional protein. Mutations in any of the classes 2 to 5 display a broad range of phenotypic effects making prediction of the clinical course of a patient impossible simply based on mutation classification. Moreover, the potential of a mutation to contribute to the phenotype depends not only on its nature, localisation in the gene and molecular mechanism, but also on its interaction with the second mutated CFTR allele as well as on disease modifiers.

Table 1.1 summarizes the 23 most common CF-causing mutations worldwide and presents their transcriptional/translational consequences, localization in the gene and classification as well as their allele frequencies in CF patients of different ethnicities. Testing for these 23 mutations detects 80% and 70% of CF alleles in Caucasian and Mediterranean populations, respectively, whereas the detection rate in CF patients of South American, African or Middle East origin is only around 60%. The G542X mutation is most common in Mediterranean and South American countries, the N1303K mutation in Mediterranean countries and the Middle East. On the other hand, A455E is only detectable in Caucasians and R560T only in Caucasians and Africans.

Table 1.2 presents additional 21 variants from CFTR2 with a frequency of ≥0.1% and originating mainly from Caucasians and Mediterranean populations. An analysis of these 21 variants detects about a further 4% of CF alleles in these populations.

Table 1.2 demonstrates how variable even the common *CFTR* mutation frequencies are across Europe. Besides F508del, there are several other *CFTR* mutations that appear to be the oldest alleles and have had the longest time to spread. For example, G542X is supposed to be associated with the ancient Phoenicians, N1303K with the ancient Mediterranean populations and G551D with the ancient Celtic tribes (Bobadilla et al., 2002). Another region of interest is Reunion Island which shows high frequencies of G551D and 3120+1G>A correlating to the 27% European and 40% African origins of the founders of this island. Further population specific mutations are: W1282X associated with the Ashkenazi Jews, 394delTT present at a high frequency in the countries around the Baltic Sea, *CFTR*dele2,3 common in regions of Central and Eastern Europe with a Slavic origin, and the 3905insT of Swiss origin.

Table 1.3 shows that 10 mutations per country account on average for 84.5% of the total number of CF chromosomes in Northern Europe and for 74.7% in Southern Europe. Moreover, the spectrum of the 10 mutations includes on average 8 of the worldwide most common 23 mutations in Central and North Europe, but only 6 of these 23 mutations in the South.

In conclusion, the frequency of most *CFTR* mutations is highly variable and depends on the ethnic and geographic background of a population. Furthermore, classification of mutations is not possible only based on the alteration within the gene, but needs additional examinations on transcript and protein level. Therefore, crucial requirements for successful mutation specific therapeutic approaches are: early and reliable genotyping of the CF patients as well as careful functional characterization and classification of the individual mutations. Nowadays, an early diagnosis can be made in the majority of cases by newborn screening, which significantly increases the quality of life and life expec-

Legacy name	cDNA position	Amino acid position	Effect on transcript/ protein level	Localization	Class	Caucasian	Mediter-ranean	South American	African	Middle East
G85E	c.254G>A	p.Gly85Glu	Missense	E3	II	0.23	0.56	0.73	0.03	0.40
R117H	c.350G>A	p.Arg117His	Missense	E4	IV	1.58	0.54	0.02	0.03	0.62
621+1G>T	c.489+1G>T	-	Splicesite	I4	I	0.63	1.31	0.16	0.37	0.00
711+1G>T	c.579+1G>T	-	Splicesite	I5	I	0.19	0.58	0.05	0.45	0.53
R334W	c.1000C>T	p.Arg334Trp	Missense	E8(7)	IV	0.15	1.13	0.90	0.57	0.74
R347P	c.1040G>C	p.Arg347Pro	Missense	E8(7)	IV	0.35	0.27	0.02	0.03	0.00
A455E	c.1364C>A	p.Ala455Glu	Missense	E10(9)	V	0.26	0.00	0.00	0.00	0.00
I507del	c.1519_1521 delATC	p.Ile507del	Inframe	E11(10)	II	0.31	0.32	0.23	0.87	0.00
F508del	c.1521_1523 delCTT	p.Phe508del	Inframe	E11(10)	II	65.7	48.5	47.5	41.0	21.7
1717-1G>A	c.1585-1G>A	-	Splicesite	I11(10)	I	0.75	0.85	0.32	0.67	0.15
G542X	c.1624G>T	p.Gly542*	Nonsense	E12(11)	I	2.27	5.28	5.33	1.03	1.93
G551D	c.1652G>A	p.Gly551Asp	Missense	E12(11)	III	2.07	0.20	0.14	0.93	0.00
R553X	c.1657C>T	p.Arg553*	Nonsense	E12(11)	I	1.22	0.54	0.51	1.10	0.32
R560T	c.1679G>C	p.Arg560Thr	Missense	E12(11)	III	0.33	0.00	0.00	0.23	0.00
1898+1G>A	c.1766+1G>A	-	Splicesite	I13(12)	I	0.14	0.13	0.07	0.05	0.47
2184delA	c.2052delA	p.Lys684Asn fs*38	Frameshift	E14(13)	I	0.13	0.12	0.02	0.05	1.62
2789+5 G>A	c.2657+5G>A	-	Splicesite, alternative	I16(14b)	V	0.21	1.16	0.21	0.00	1.46
3120+1 G>A	c.2988+1G>A	-	Splicesite	I18(16)	I	0.29	0.24	0.28	10.2	6.40
R1162X	c.3484C>T	p.Arg1162*	Nonsense	E22(19)	I	0.46	2.65	0.96	0.40	0.35
3659delC	c.3528delC	p.Lys1177Serfs*15	Frameshift	E22(19)	I	0.44	0.00	0.09	0.05	0.00
3849+10kbC>T	c.3717+12191C>T	-	Splicesite, alternative	I22(19)	V	0.29	0.21	0.41	0.07	1.15
W1282X	c.3846G>A	p.Trp1282*	Nonsense	E23(20)	I	0.87	1.07	1.13	0.07	13.0
N1303K	c.3909C>G	p.Asn1303Lys	Missense	E24(21)	II	1.17	3.78	1.65	0.30	8.76
Detection rate%						**80.04**	**69.44**	**60.73**	**58.50**	**59.6**

Table 1.1: The ACMG recommended testing of the 23 most common CF causing mutations worldwide: Localization, classification and allele frequencies (%) in CF patients by major ethnic groups (Clancy et al., 2014; Perez et al., 2007; WHO report, 2004). E = exon, I = intron, () = old nomenclature. Caucasian = CF patients from North-, East- and Central Europe, North America and Australia. Mediterranean = CF patients from Spain, Italy, Greece, Turkey. South American = CF patients from Argentina, Brazil, Chile, Colombia, Costa Rica, Mexico, Uruguay and Venezuela. African = Afro-American CF patients. Middle East = CF patients from Iran, Israel, Jordan and Lebanon. R117H: According to CFTR2 (www.cftr2.org), the R117H variant is no longer considered to be a priori causative of CF, but rather a variant of varying clinical consequences (VCC).

tancy. As far as genotyping is concerned, new technological developments such as high-throughput sequencing allow to analyze in a short time the whole *CFTR* gene and to detect all known CF variants, including deep intronic (such as 1811+1.6kb A>G, 3849+10kbC>T, c.3874-4522A>G; Bergougnoux A et al., 2019) and population-specific ones, as well as new ones, which is a great advantage over the mutation-specific diagnostic tests commercially available (Pereira et al., 2019).

The database of the Cystic Fibrosis Genetic Analysis Consortium (CFGAC; www.genet.sickkids.on.ca) was last updated in April 2011 and is still online, but the database CFTR2 (www.cftr2.org) continues to update expert-reviewed functional and clinical information on *CFTR* mutations. The domestic database *CFTR*-France (Claustres et al., 2017) compiles more than 900 sequence variants from over 5,000 individuals and is currently the most authoritative resource of up-to-date information about *CFTR* genetics. *CFTR*-France (https://cftr.iurc.montp.inserm.fr/cgi-bin/home.cgi?) compiles any category of variations (disease-causing, non disease-causing and variants of unknown clinical significance) that have been identified in the following situations:

- Patients affected with CF
- Patients presenting milder phenotypes named *CFTR*-related disorders (*CFTR*-RD)
- Fetuses with abnormal ultrasonography (echogenic bowel, ...)
- Newborns with pending or inconclusive diagnosis
- Asymptomatic individuals carrying at least one sequence variation on each *CFTR* gene (i.e. carrying two variations in *trans*).

Legacy name	cDNA position	Amino acid position	Effect on transcript/ protein level	CFTR localization	Class*	CFTR2 frequency
CFTRdele2,3	c.54-5940_273+10250del2	p.Ser18Argfs	Frameshift	E2+3	I	0.29
E60X	c.178G>T	p.Glu60*	Nonsense	E3	I	0.21
P67L	c.200C>T	p.Pro67Leu	Missense	E3	III	0.17
394delTT	c.262_263delTT	p.Leu88Ilefs*22	Frameshift	E3	I	0.22
R117C	c.349C>T	p.Arg117Cys	Missense	E4	III	0.10
L206W	c.617T>G	p.Leu206Trp	Missense	E6(6a)	III	0.23
1078delT	c.948delT	p.Phe316Leufs*12	Frameshift	E8(7)	I	0.13
1154insTC	c.1021_1022dupTC	p.Phe342Hisfs*28	Frameshift	E8(7)	I	0.15
R347H	c.1040G>A	p.Arg347His	Missense	E8(7)	III	0.14
Q493X	c.1477C>T	p.Gln493*	Nonsense	E11(10)	I	0.21
V520F	c.1558G>T	p.Val520Phe	Missense	E11(10)	II	0.11
S549N	c.1646G>A	p.Ser549Asn	Missense	E12(11)	III	0.14
2183AA->G	c.2051_2052delAAinsG	p.Lys684Serfs*38	Frameshift	E14(13)	I	0.38
2184insA	c.2052dupA	p.Gln685Thrfs*4	Frameshift	E14(13)	I	0.23
S945L	c.2834C>T	p.Ser945Leu	Missense	E17(15)	III	0.12
3272-26A->G	c.3140-26A>G	-	Splicesite, alternative	I19(17a)	V	0.33
R1066C	3196C>T	p.Arg1066Cys	Missense	E20(17b)	II	0.15
Y1092X	c.3276C>A or C>G	p.Tyr1092*	Nonsense	E20(17b)	I	0.16
M1101K	c.3302T>A	p.Met1101Lys	Missense	E20(17b)	II	0.17
R1158X	c.3472C>T	p.Arg1158*	Nonsense	E22(19)	I	0.13
3905insT	c.3773dupT	p.Leu1258PhefsX7	Frameshift	E23(20)	I	0.15

Table 1.2: Another 21 variants with a frequency of ≥0.1% based on the information from 71,018 patients (142,036 alleles) with cystic fibrosis variants from the United States, Canada, and Europe (Source: CFTR2, September 2021; https://cftr2/org). * = Classification according to Villa-Nova Pereira et al., 2019. E = exon, I = intron, () = old nomenclature.

	Chromo-somes n	*CFTR* mutations (legacy names) and their frequencies in %										Detection rate %
Northern Europe												
Belarus[1]	238	**F508del** 60.9	Dele2,3 5.9	**N1303K** 2.8	**G542X** 1.3	**W1282X** 0.8						**71.7**
Belgium[1]	392	**F508del** 76.0	**G542X** 3.8	**N1303K** 2.8	**1717-1** **G>A** 1.8	E60X 1.5	S1251N 1.5	2183AA >G 1.3	**W1282X** 1.0	W401X 0.5	**A455E** 0.5	**90.7**
Denmark[1]	825	**F508del** 86.7	394delTT 1.9	**N1303K** 1.3	**3659del** **C** 1.0	**621+1** **G>T** 0.7	**G542X** 0.6	E60X 0.5	**R117H** 0.5	**1717-1** **G>A** 0.5	**W1282X** 0.5	**93.7**
France[1]	7420	**F508del** 67.2	**G542X** 2.9	**N1303K** 2.1	**1717-1** **G>A** 1.3	**G551D** 1.0	**2789+5** **G>A** 1.0	**R553X** 0.9	**W1282X** 0.9	1078del T 0.7	**I507del** 0.7	**78.7**
Germany[1]	2324	**F508del** 70.2	**N1303K** 2.5	**G542X** 2.1	**G551D** 2.0	**R553X** 1.5	Dele2,3 1.5	**R347P** 1.4	**1717-1** **G>A** 1.2	**3849+10** **C>T** 1.1	**R117H** 0.9	**84.4**
Ireland[1]	1318	**F508del** 76.4	**G551D** 6.7	**R117H** 3.0	**R560T** 2.4	**621+1** **G>T** 1.6	**I507del** 0.8	**1717-1** **G>A** 0.7	**G542X** 0.6	1461ins4 0.4	**N1303K** 0.4	**93.0**
Lithuania[1]	118	**F508del** 55.9	**R553X** 3.4	**N1303K** 1.7	Dele2,3 1.7	G314R 0.8	**W1282X** 0.8					**64.3**
Nether-lands[1]	804	**F508del** 79.2	**A455E** 2.6	**G542X** 1.6	**1717-1** **G>A** 1.5	S1251N 1.5	**R553X** 1.4	**R1162X** 1.1	3272-26 A>G 0.9	**W1282X** 0.9	**N1303K** 0.8	**91.5**
Norway[1]	282	**F508del** 70.9	394delTT 3.9	R117C 2.8	4005+2 T>C 2.5	**R117H** 2.1	**3659del** **C** 1.8	**G551D** 1.4	**G542X** 0.7	**N1303K** 0.7		**86.8**
Poland[2]	1476	**F508del** 54.5	Dele2,3 4.5	**3849+10** **C>T** 3.9	2012del T 1.8	**1717-1** **G>A** 1.8	**G542X** 1.7	**R347P** 1.6	**N1303K** 1.2	**R553X** 0.9	**W1282X** 0.6	**72.5**
Russia[1]	668	**F508del** 53.4	Dele2,3 5.7	**N1303K** 2.7	2143del T 2.0	2184ins A 2.0	**G542X** 1.7	**W1282X** 1.7	**3849+10** **C>T** 1.1	**R334W** 0.8	394delTT 0.6	**71.7**
Sweden[1]	920	**F508del** 66.6	394delTT 7.5	**3659del** **C** 6.2	R117C 0.8	E60X 0.4	1112del T 0.4	R764X 0.4	**R117H** 0.3	**621+1** **G>T** 0.3		**82.9**
UK[1]	9804	**F508del** 75.4	**G551D** 3.1	**G542X** 1.7	**621+1** **G>T** 0.9	**1717-1** **G>A** 0.6	**R117H** 0.5	**R553X** 0.5	**1898+1** **G>A** 0.5	**N1303K** 0.5	**R560T** 0.4	**84.1**
Ukraine[1]	580	**F508del** 50.0	**N1303K** 2.4	Dele2,3 1.0	**W1282X** 0.5							**53.9**

	Chromo-somes n	*CFTR* mutations (legacy names) and their frequencies in %										Detection rate %
Southern Europe												
Albania[1]	146	**F508del** 69.9	**G85E** 0.7	C276X 0.7	R1070Q 0.7							**72.0**
Austria[1]	824	**F508del** 65.2	**G542X** 4.2	**R1162X** 2.7	**G551D** 1.5	Dele2,3 1.5	**R553X** 1.2	457TAT >G 1.1	**R347P** 0.8	2183AA >G 0.8	**R117H** 0.7	**79.7**
Bulgaria[1]	506	**F508del** 63.8	**N1303K** 4.7	**G542X** 3.8	**R347P** 2.0	1677del TA 1.8	R1070Q 1.6	Q220X 1.2	**3849+10** **C>T** 1.2	**W1282X** 1.0	G1244V 1.0	**82.1**
Croatia[1]	276	**F508del** 64.5	**G542X** 3.3	**N1303K** 2.9	**G551D** 1.1	**3849+10** **C>T** 0.7						**72.5**
Czech Rep.[3]	1200	**F508del** 67.4	Dele2,3 5.7	**G551D** 2.9	**N1303K** 2.4	**G542X** 2.0	**3849+10** **C>T** 1.7	**1898+1** **G>A** 1.4	**R347P** 0.9	2143del T 0.9	3272-26 A>G 0.7	**86.0**
Greece[1]	1006	**F508del** 53.8	**621+1** **G>T** 6.6	**G542X** 4.1	**N1303K** 2.5	**2789+5** **G>A** 1.5	E822X 1.4	2183AA >G 1.2	R1158X 0.9	**R334W** 0.8	R1070Q 0.8	**73.6**
Hungary[1]	1022	**F508del** 52.7	**G542X** 2.2	Dele2,3 1.8	**N1303K** 1.1	**R553X** 0.9	**W1282X** 0.5	2184ins A 0.3				**58.4**
Italy[1]	3873	**F508del** 52.0	**N1303K** 6.1	**G542X** 5.2	2183AA >G 2.3	**1717-1** **G>A** 2.2	**R1162X** 1.7	**W1282X** 1.5	**2789+5** **G>A** 1.4	**R553X** 1.1	**R347P** 0.8	**74.3**
Macedo-nia[1]	226	**F508del** 61.1	**G542X** 4.9	**N1303K** 2.2	**621+1** **G>T** 1.3	Dele2,3 1.3	457TAT >G 0.9	711+3 A>G 0.9	2184ins A 0.9	3849 G>A 0.9	V1397E 0.9	**74.0**
Portugal[1]	494	**F508del** 59.3	A561E 3.2	**R334W** 2.8	R1066C 2.8	**G542X** 2.6	**G85E** 2.2	**N1303K** 1.8	G576A 1.4	**711+1** **G>T** 1.0	3272-26 A>G 1.0	**78.1**
Romania[1]	153	**F508del** 58.8	**G542X** 2.6	**W1282X** 2.6	Dele2,3 2.0	457TAT >G 0.7	**R117H** 0.7	**621+1** **G>T** 0.7	**R334W** 0.7			**68.8**
Serbia[1]	622	**F508del** 66.1	**G542X** 3.4	**621+1** **G>T** 1.0	S466X 0.5	525delT 0.3	**G551D** 0.3	**2789+5** **G>A** 0.3	R1070Q 0.3	**N1303K** 0.3		**72.5**
Slovakia[3]	856	**F508del** 66.8	**3849+10** **C>T** 4.3	**G542X** 4.1	Dele2,3 2.3	**N1303K** 2.0	2184ins A 1.6	**R347P** 1.1	2143del T 1.1	**R553X** 0.9	**W1282X** 0.5	**84.7**
Slovenia[1]	132	**F508del** 52.3	**R1162X** 3.0	Q552X 1.5	Q685X 1.5	3905ins T 1.5	Dele2,3 1.5	S4X 0.8	457TAT >G 0.8	**R347P** 0.8	**G542X** 0.8	**64.5**

	Chromosomes n	*CFTR* mutations (legacy names) and their frequencies in %										Detection rate %
Spain[4]	1634	**F508del** 51.7	**G542X** 7.7	**N1303K** 2.9	1811+1.6 A>G 1.8	**R334W** 1.8	L206W 1.6	**711+1 G>T** 1.6	Q890X 1.4	**R1162X** 1.3	**2789+5 G>A** 1.2	**73.0**
Switzerland[5]	1164	**F508del** 65.2	3905ins T 4.8	**R553X** 3.8	**1717-1 G>A** 3.7	**G542X** 1.8	**W1282X** 1.6	**N1303K** 1.6	R347H 1.1	2347del G 0.8	**R117H** 0.8	**85.2**
Turkey[1]	246	**F508del** 22.0	1677del TA 4.5	**G542X** 2.9	2183AA >G 2.9	**N1303K** 2.4	E92K 2.0	**2789+5 G>A** 2.0	R347H 1.6	2043del G 1.6	G85E 1.2	**43.1**

Table 1.3: European *CFTR* mutation spectrum: The 4 to 10 most common mutations and their detection rate. **Bold** mutation names = included in the 23 most common CF-causing mutations recommended by the ACMG. **R117H** = variant with varying clinical consequence (VCC) depending on the poly-T tract in intron 9 of the *CFTR* gene. R117H in *cis* with 5T will likely act as a disease-causing variant whereas in combination with 7T it is unlikely to cause CF but may result in male infertility. Thus, R117H needs always to be interpreted in the context of the poly-T tract. [1] WHO report 2004. [2] Zietkiewicz et al., 2014. [3] Krenkova et al., 2013. [4] Alonso et al., 2006. [5] Gallati et al., 2009.

Within this context, the team of the database addressed the important clinical issues of the penetrance of *CFTR* sequence variants (Boussaroque et al., 2020) and the risk of over-classifying variants as CF-causing when consulting clinical databases (Boussaroque et al., 2019).

Moreover, candidate modifier genes, regulatory loci, epigenetic profiles and trans-regulators refine genotype-phenotype correlations at the individual level that contribute to the large phenotypic variability between patients with CF, even when they carry identical CFTR variants (Raynal and Corvol, 2020). In particular, pharmacogenetic factors may modify the clinical response to the hydrophobic CFTR modulators that give rise to multiple drug-drug interactions during biotransformation in the liver (☞ Chapter 5.2.).

1.6. Molecular pathology of *CFTR* mutations

Burkhard Tümmler

Based primarily on the examination in heterologous expression systems *in vitro*, *CFTR* mutations have been assigned to six classes (Welsh and Smith, 1993; ☞ Figure 1.10):

- Class 1: absent or defective synthesis of CFTR protein
- Class 2: defective posttranslational maturation and/or trafficking
- Class 3: defective regulation of the ion channel (gating mutations)
- Class 4: altered channel properties (open probability, open time, ion selectivity, conductance)
- Class 5: decreased production of wild type CFTR
- Class 6: reduced stability of CFTR (reduced half-life)

Information about the phenotype of individual mutations and its impact on CF disease is compiled in the CFTR2 database (http://www.cftr2.org; Sosnay et al., 2013). Patients who harbour two class 1, 2, 3, or 6 *CFTR* alleles typically suffer from the whole spectrum of CF disease including exocrine pancreatic insufficiency. Individuals with two *CFTR* mutations in trans who harbour at least one class 4 or 5 *CFTR* allele are affected by milder forms of CFTR-associated disease; i.e. CF with exocrine pancreatic sufficiency or CFTR-related disorders such as bronchiectasis or congenital bilateral absence of the vas deferens (CBAVD; ☞ Figures 1.8+1.10).

1.6.1. Deletions, frame-shift mutations and stop mutations

Large deletions, frame-shifts and stop mutations normally belong to class 1. In most cases the mutations lead to the synthesis of mRNA transcripts with a premature stop codon which are subject to nonsense mediated decay. Moreover, exon skipping (p.Glu60Ter, p.Arg75Ter, p.Arg553Ter) or the activation of cryptic splice sites may be induced by a stop mutation (Hull et al., 1994; Will et al., 1994; 1995). No CFTR protein was detectable in CF epithelial tissue of index cases who were homo-

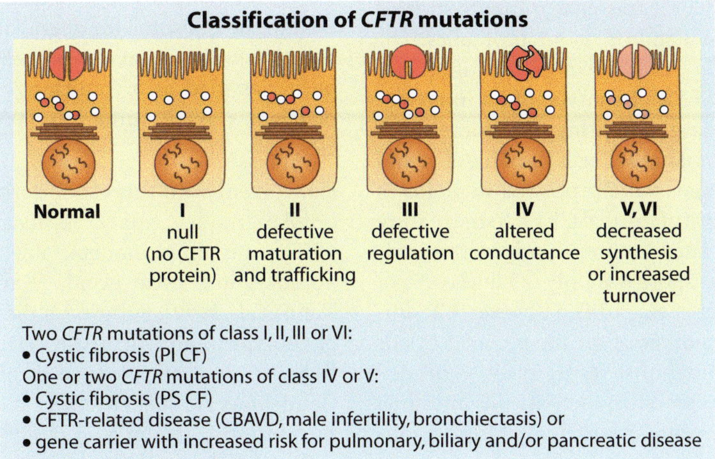

Figure 1.10: Classification of *CFTR* mutations.

zygous for the stop mutations p.Gly542Ter or p.Arg553Ter or large deletion cftrdele2,3(21 kb; Kälin et al., 1999). Thus the most common class I mutations are null alleles. The exceptions are stop mutations close to the C-terminus which give rise to short-lived truncated CFTR isoforms (class 6 mutation: p.Leu1399Ter, p.Gln1412Ter; Haardt et al., 1999) or singular cases of CFTR mutants of almost normal function (p.Ser1455Ter, Mickle et al., 1998; p.Glu831Ter, Hinzpeter et al., 2010).

1.6.2. Splice mutations

Splice mutations belong to either class 1 or class 5. If the nucleotide substitution affects an obligatorily conserved position in the donor or acceptor splice site, the adjacent exon will not be recognized which leads to exon skipping and sometimes also to the activation of a cryptic splice site. Nucleotide substitutions at other positions will typically results in both normal and aberrant CFTR mRNA isoforms. Absolute and relative quantities of correct and aberrant transcript vary among different tissues and patients resulting in a broad heterogeneity of disease manifestation among individuals with class 5 mutations such as c.2657+5G>A, c.3140-26A>G, c.3717+12191C>T or the T_5-allele c.1210-12T(5) of the splice acceptor site in intron 9 (Nissim-Rafinia and Kerem, 2006).

1.6.3. Missense mutations

Our knowledge about the phenotype of CFTR missense mutants is mainly based on analyses in heterologous expression systems (e.g., van Goor et al., 2014). Most CFTR missense mutants showed some class 2, class 3 and/or class 4 anomalies. The data generated *in vitro*, however, do often not match with the CFTR phenotype of an index patient who is homozygous for this mutation. For example, in recombinant FRT cells the Glu92Lys and Met1101Lys mutants were processed in yields of only 1.9% and 0.3% of normal CFTR to the mature complex glycosylated isoform and correspondingly chloride transport was only 0.3 and 0.0% of normal (van Goor et al., 2014). However, CF subjects who are homozygous for the p.Glu92 Lys or p.Met1101Lys mutations, respectively, exhibited residual chloride secretory activity in intestinal current measurements or residual chloride conductance in nasal potential difference measurements (☞ Chapter 2.; Stanke et al., 2008). According to the author's experience the phenotype is more variable among class 2 than among class 3 or class 4 missense mutations. For example, a consistent phenotype of residual chloride secretion was observed in a cohort of CF patients who are compound heterozygous for the class 3 gating mutant p.Gly551Asp CFTR, which is properly targeted in wild-type amounts to the cell surface (Graeber et al., 2015).

1.6.4. The major mutation p.Phe508del

Phenylalanine508 resides on the surface of NBD1 of CFTR (Riordan, 2008). Deletion of Phe508 exerts only minor local effects on NBD1 structure around position 508 (Lewis et al., 2010), but it precludes the proper assembly between the cytoplasmic and membrane-integrated domains of CFTR including interactions between NBD1 and the fourth intracellular loop of CFTR within the second membrane spanning domain (Lukacs and Verkman, 2012; Thibodeau et al., 2010; Okiyoneda et al., 2013). *In vitro* most of the newly synthesized Phe508del CFTR fails to adopt a wild-type fold in the endoplasmic reticulum (ER) and is targeted to ER-associated degradation (Ward et al., 1995). Chaperone-assisted modulation of the folding of the nascent protein (Wang et al., 2006) or biosynthesis at temperatures below 30°C (Denning et al., 1992) can rescue Phe508del CFTR. However, any Phe508del CFTR protein that reaches the cell surface remains thermally unstable, capable of only partial chloride channel activity (Dalemans et al., 1991), and is rapidly endocytosed and finally delivered to the lysosome for degradation (Gentzsch et al., 2004). In summary, p.Phe508del *CFTR* has been classified as a trafficking- and processing-deficient class 2 mutation (Welsh and Smith, 1993).

Concurrent with this classification inferred from cellular models, only mislocalized Phe508del CFTR was immunodetectable in p.Phe508del homozygotes' sweat glands (Kartner et al., 1992; Kälin et al., 1999). Reports on the Phe508del CFTR phenotype in human airways (Dupuit et al., 1995; Kälin et al., 1999; Penque et al., 2000; Sermet-Gaudelus et al., 2002; Kreda et al., 2005) and in human intestine (Kälin et al., 1999; Bronsveld et al., 2001, Mall et al., 2004) are inconsistent. Taking a set of high-affinity anti-CFTR antibodies no Phe

508del CFTR mature protein or function could be detected (Mall et al., 2004; Kreda et al., 2005), whereas mature complex-glycosylated Phe508del CFTR (Kälin et al., 1999) and residual Phe508del-CFTR-mediated chloride conductance (Bronsveld et al., 2001) had been described before in p.Phe 508del homozygous people with CF. To resolve the molecular pathology of Phe508del CFTR, the author's laboratory characterized freshly excised Phe 508del CFTR homozygous rectal mucosa by bio-electric measurement of the basic defect and Phe 508del CFTR protein by metabolic labelling or immunoblot (van Barneveld et al., 2010; Stanke et al., 2022). The majority of investigated p.Phe508 del homozygous subjects expressed low amounts of glycoform C of Phe508del CFTR (☞ Chapter 2.5.) and low residual Phe508del CFTR-mediated chloride secretory activity in the rectal mucosa (van Barneveld et al., 2010; Stanke et al., 2022). In summary, some Phe508del CFTR can exit the ER to be delivered to the apical epithelial membrane, which can be boosted by CFTR correctors (☞ Chapter 5.).

1.7. References

Abdullah LH, Evans JR, Wang TT, Ford AA, Makhov AM, Nguyen K, Coakley RD, Griffith JD, Davis CW, Ballard ST, Kesimer M. Defective postsecretory maturation of MUC5B mucin in cystic fibrosis airways. JCI Insight. 2017;2:e89752. doi: 10.1172/jci.insight.89752.

Al Salmani MK, Sondo E, Balut C, Sheppard DN, Singh AK, Pedemonte N. Molecular Physiology and Pharmacology of the Cystic Fibrosis Transmembrane Conductance Regulator. In: Studies of Epithelial Transporters and Ion Channels, Physiology in Health and Disease, Second Edition, Volume 3, Chapter 16, pages 605-670, 2020, Eds Hamilton KL, Devor DC, American Physiological Society/Springer-Verlag.

Aleksandrov L, Aleksandrov AA, Chang X-B, Riordan JR. The first nucleotide binding domain of cystic fibrosis transmembrane conductance regulator is a site of stable nucleotide interaction, whereas the second is a site of rapid turnover. J Biol Chem 2002;277:15419-15425. doi: 10.1074/jbc.M111713200.

Aleksandrov AA, Kota P, Aleksandrov LA, He L, Jensen T, Cui L, Gentzsch M, Dokholyan NV, Riordan JR. Regulatory insertion removal restores maturation, stability and function of ΔF508 CFTR. J Mol Biol 2010;401:194-210. doi: 10.1016/j.jmb.2010.06.019.

Alonso MJ, Heine-Suñer D, Calvo M, Rosell J, Giménez J, Ramos MD, Telleria JJ, Palacio A, Estivill X, Casals T. Spectrum of mutations in the CFTR gene in cystic fibrosis patients of Spanish ancestry. Ann Hum Genet. 2007; 71:194-201. doi: 10.1111/j.1469-1809.2006.00310.x.

Amaral MD, Farinha CM. Rescuing mutant CFTR: a multi-task approach to a better outcome in treating cystic fibrosis. Curr Pharm Des. 2013;19:3497-508. doi: 10.2174/13816128113199990318.

Anderson MP, Gregory RJ, Thompson S, Souza DW, Paul S, Mulligan RC, Smith AE, Welsh MJ. Demonstration that CFTR is a chloride channel by alteration of its anion selectivity. Science. 1991;253:202-5. doi: 10.1126/science.1712984.

Bai Y, Li M, Hwang T-C. Structural basis for the channel function of a degraded ABC transporter, CFTR (ABCC7). J Gen Physiol 2011;138:495-507. doi: 10.1085/jgp.201110705.

Barry PJ, Taylor-Cousar JL. Triple combination cystic fibrosis transmembrane conductance regulator modulator therapy in the real world - opportunities and challenges. Curr Opin Pulm Med. 2021;27:554-66. doi: 10.1097/MCP.0000000000000819.

Bell SC, Mall MA, Gutierrez H, Macek M, Madge S, Davies JC, Burgel PR, Tullis E, Castaños C, Castellani C, Byrnes CA, Cathcart F, Chotirmall SH, Cosgriff R, Eichler I, Fajac I, Goss CH, Drevinek P, Farrell PM, Gravelle AM, Havermans T, Mayer-Hamblett N, Kashirskaya N, Kerem E, Mathew JL, McKone EF, Naehrlich L, Nasr SZ, Oates GR, O'Neill C, Pypops U, Raraigh KS, Rowe SM, Southern KW, Sivam S, Stephenson AL, Zampoli M, Ratjen F. The future of cystic fibrosis care: a global perspective. Lancet Respir Med. 2020;8:65-124. doi: 10.1016/S2213-2600(19)30337-6.

Berdiev BK, Qadri YJ, Benos DJ. Assessment of the CFTR and ENaC association. Mol Biosyst. 2009;5:123-7. doi: 10.1039/b810471a.

Bergougnoux A, Délétang K, Pommier A, Varilh J, Houriez F, Altieri JP, Koenig M, Férec C, Claustres M, Lalau G, Bienvenu T, Audrézet MP, Pagin A, Girodon E, Raynal C, Taulan-Cadars M. Functional characterization and phenotypic spectrum of three recurrent disease-causing deep intronic variants of the CFTR gene. J Cyst Fibros. 2019;18:468-475. doi: 10.1016/j.jcf.2018.10.012.

Betapudi B, Aleem A, Kothadia JP. Cystic fibrosis and liver disease. 2021. In: StatPearls [Internet]. Treasure Island (FL): StatPearls Publishing. PMID: 32310546. Bookshelf ID: NBK556086

Blanchard AC, Waters VJ. Microbiology of cystic fibrosis airway disease. Semin Respir Crit Care Med. 2019;40: 727-736. doi: 10.1055/s-0039-1698464.

Bobadilla JL, Macek M Jr, Fine JP, Farrell PM. Cystic fibrosis: a worldwide analysis of CFTR mutations—correlation with incidence data and application to screening.

Hum Mutat. 2002;19:575-606. doi: 10.1002/humu.10041.

Boucher RC. Airway surface dehydration in cystic fibrosis: pathogenesis and therapy. Annu Rev Med. 2007;58: 157-170. doi: 10.1146/annurev.med.58.071905.105316.

Boussaroque A, Bergougnoux A, Raynal C, Audrézet MP, Sasorith S, Férec C, Bienvenu T, Girodon E. Pitfalls in the interpretation of CFTR variants in the context of incidental findings. Hum Mutat. 2019;40:2239-2246. doi: 10.1002/humu.23884.

Boussaroque A, Audrézet MP, Raynal C, Sermet-Gaudelus I, Bienvenu T, Férec C, Bergougnoux A, Lopez M, Scotet V, Munck A, Girodon E. Penetrance is a critical parameter for assessing the disease liability of CFTR variants. J Cyst Fibros. 2020;19:949-954. doi: 10.1016/j.jcf.2020.03.019.

Bozoky Z, Krzeminski M, Muhandiram R, Birtley JR, Al-Zahrani A, Thomas PJ, Frizzell RA, Ford RC, Forman-Kay JD. Regulatory R region of the CFTR chloride channel is a dynamic integrator of phospho-dependent intra- and intermolecular interactions. Proc Natl Acad Sci U S A. 2013;110:E4427-36. doi: 10.1073/pnas.1315104110.

Bronsveld I, Mekus F, Bijman J, Ballmann M, de Jonge HR, Laabs U, Halley DJ, Ellemunter H, Mastella G, Thomas S, Veeze HJ, Tümmler B. Chloride conductance and genetic background modulate the cystic fibrosis phenotype of Delta F508 homozygous twins and siblings. J Clin Invest. 2001;108:1705-15. doi: 10.1172/JCI12108.

Cai ZW, Liu J, Li HY, Sheppard DN. Targeting F508del-CFTR to develop rational new therapies for cystic fibrosis. Acta Pharmacol Sin. 2011;32:693-701.

Chang XB, Tabcharani JA, Hou YX, Jensen TJ, Kartner N, Alon N, Hanrahan JW, Riordan JR. Protein kinase A (PKA) still activates CFTR chloride channel after mutagenesis of all 10 PKA consensus phosphorylation sites. J Biol Chem 1993;268:11304-11311.

Chen JH, Stoltz DA, Karp PH, Ernst SE, Pezzulo AA, Moninger TO, Rector MV, Reznikov LR, Launspach JL, Chaloner K, Zabner J, Welsh MJ. Loss of anion transport without increased sodium absorption characterizes newborn porcine cystic fibrosis airway epithelia. Cell 2010; 143: 911-923. doi: 10.1016/j.cell.2010.11.029.

Chen JH, Xu W, Sheppard DN. Altering intracellular pH reveals the kinetic basis of intraburst gating in the CFTR Cl^- channel. J Physiol. 2017;595:1059-76. doi: 10.1113/JP273205.

Chen X, Zhu S, Zhenin M, Xu W, Bose SJ, Wong MP, Leung GPH, Senderowitz H, Chen JH. A defective flexible loop contributes to the processing and gating defects of the predominant cystic fibrosis-causing mutation. FASEB J. 2019;33:5126-42. doi: 10.1096/fj.201801218RR.

Cheng SH, Rich DP, Marshall J, Gregory RJ, Welsh MJ, Smith AE. Phosphorylation of the R domain by cAMP-dependent protein kinase regulates the CFTR chloride channel. Cell. 1991; 66:1027-36. doi: 10.1016/0092-8674(91)90446-6.

Csanaìdy LS, Chan KW, Nairn AC, Gadsby DC. Functional roles of nonconserved structural segments in CFTR's NH_2-terminal nucleotide binding domain. J Gen Physiol 2005;125:43-55. doi: 10.1085/jgp.200409174.

Csanády L, Vergani P, Gadsby DC. Structure, gating, and regulation of the CFTR anion channel. Physiol Rev 2019; 99:707-738. doi: 10.1152/physrev.00007.2018.

Choi JY, Muallem D, Kiselyov K, Lee MG, Thomas PJ, Muallem S. Aberrant CFTR-dependent HCO_3^- transport in mutations associated with cystic fibrosis. Nature. 2001;410: 94-97. doi: 10.1038/35065099.

Claustres M, Thèze C, des Georges M, Baux D, Girodon E, Bienvenu T, Audrezet MP, Dugueperoux I, Férec C, Lalau G, Pagin A, Kitzis A, Thoreau V, Gaston V, Bieth E, Malinge MC, Reboul MP, Fergelot P, Lemonnier L, Mekki C, Fanen P, Bergougnoux A, Sasorith S, Raynal C, Bareil C. *CFTR*-France, a national relational patient database for sharing genetic and phenotypic data associated with rare CFTR variants. Hum Mutat. 2017;38: 1297-1315. doi: 10.1002/humu.23276.

Cystic Fibrosis Genetic Analysis Consortium. http://www.genet.sickkids.on.ca/cftr/app

Dalemans W, Barbry P, Champigny G, Jallat S, Dott K, Dreyer D, Crystal RG, Pavirani A, Lecocq JP, Lazdunski M. Altered chloride ion channel kinetics associated with the delta F508 cystic fibrosis mutation. Nature. 1991;354: 526-8. doi: 10.1038/354526a0.

Denning GM, Anderson MP, Amara JF, Marshall J, Smith AE, Welsh MJ. Processing of mutant cystic fibrosis transmembrane conductance regulator is temperature-sensitive. Nature. 1992;358:761-4. doi: 10.1038/358761a0.

Dupuit F, Kälin N, Brézillon S, Hinnrasky J, Tümmler B, Puchelle E. CFTR and differentiation markers expression in non-CF and delta F 508 homozygous CF nasal epithelium. J Clin Invest. 1995;96:1601-11. doi: 10.1172/JCI118199.

Engelhardt JF, Yankaskas JR, Ernst SA, Yang Y, Marino CR, Boucher RC, Cohn JA, Wilson JM. Submucosal glands are the predominant site of CFTR expression in the human bronchus. Nat Genet. 1992;2:240-8. doi: 10.1038/ng1192-240.

Engelhardt JF, Zepeda M, Cohn JA, Yankaskas JR, Wilson JM. Expression of the cystic fibrosis gene in adult human lung. J Clin Invest. 1994;93:737-49. doi: 10.1172/JCI117028.

Farinha CM, Canato S. From the endoplasmic reticulum to the plasma membrane: mechanisms of CFTR folding and trafficking. Cell Mol Life Sci. 2017;74:39-55. doi: 10.1007/s00018-016-2387-7.

Gallati S, Hess S, Galié-Wunder D, Berger-Menz E, Böhlen D. Cystic fibrosis transmembrane conductance regulator mutations in azoospermic and oligospermic men and their partners. Reprod Biomed Online. 2009;19:685-94. doi: 10.1016/j.rbmo.2009.09.002.

Gao X, Hwang T-C. Localizing a gate in CFTR. Proc Natl Acad Sci U. S. A. 2015;112:2461-2466. doi: 10.1073/pnas.1420676112.

Gentzsch M, Chang XB, Cui L, Wu Y, Ozols VV, Choudhury A, Pagano RE, Riordan JR. Endocytic trafficking routes of wild type and DeltaF508 cystic fibrosis transmembrane conductance regulator. Mol Biol Cell. 2004; 15:2684-96. doi: 10.1091/mbc.e04-03-0176.

Guggino WB, Stanton BA. New insights into cystic fibrosis: molecular switches that regulate CFTR. Nat Rev Mol Cell Biol. 2006;7:426-36. doi: 10.1038/nrm1949.

Gustafsson JK, Ermund A, Ambort D, Johansson ME, Nilsson HE, Thorell K, Hebert H, Sjovall H, Hansson GC. Bicarbonate and functional CFTR channel are required for proper mucin secretion and link cystic fibrosis with its mucus phenotype. J Exp Med 2012;209:1263-1272. doi:10.1084/jem.20120562

Haardt M, Benharouga M, Lechardeur D, Kartner N, Lukacs GL. C-terminal truncations destabilize the cystic fibrosis transmembrane conductance regulator without impairing its biogenesis. A novel class of mutation. J Biol Chem. 1999;274:21873-7. doi: 10.1074/jbc.274.31.21873.

Hegedûs T, Aleksandrov A, Mengos A, Cui L, Jensen TJ, Riordan JR. Role of individual R domain phosphorylation sites in CFTR regulation by protein kinase A. Biochim Biophys Acta Biomembr 2009;1788:1341-1349. doi: 10.1016/j.bbamem.2009.03.015.

Hinzpeter A, Aissat A, Sondo E, Costa C, Arous N, Gameiro C, Martin N, Tarze A, Weiss L, de Becdelièvre A, Costes B, Goossens M, Galietta LJ, Girodon E, Fanen P. Alternative splicing at a NAGNAG acceptor site as a novel phenotype modifier. PLoS Genet. 2010;6(10). doi: 10.1371/journal.pgen.1001153.

Hoegger MJ, Fischer AJ, McMenimen JD, Ostedgaard LS, Tucker AJ, Awadalla MA, Moninger TO, Michalski AS, Hoffman EA, Zabner J, Stoltz DA, Welsh MJ. Impaired mucus detachment disrupts mucociliary transport in a piglet model of cystic fibrosis. Science. 2014; 345:818-22. doi: 10.1126/science.1255825.

Hoffmann B, Elbahnsi A, Lehn P, Décout J-L, Pietrucci F, Mornon J-P, Callebaut I. Combining theoretical and experimental data to decipher CFTR 3D structures and functions. Cell Mol Life Sci 2018;75:3829-3855. doi: 10.1007/s00018-018-2835-7.

Holland IB, Cole SPC, Kuchler K, Higgins CF. ABC proteins: from bacteria to man. 2003. London, Academic Press.

Hull J, Shackleton S, Harris A. The stop mutation R553X in the *CFTR* gene results in exon skipping. Genomics. 1994;19:362-4. doi: 10.1006/geno.1994.1070.

Hwang T-C, Yeh J-T, Zhang J, Yu Y-C, Yeh H-I, Destefano S. Structural mechanisms of CFTR function and dysfunction. J Gen Physiol 2018;150:539-570. doi: 10.1085/jgp.201711946.

Kälin N, Claass A, Sommer M, Puchelle E, Tümmler B. DeltaF508 CFTR protein expression in tissues from patients with cystic fibrosis. J Clin Invest. 1999;103:1379-89. doi: 10.1172/JCI5731.

Kartner N, Augustinas O, Jensen TJ, Naismith AL, Riordan JR. Mislocalization of delta F508 CFTR in cystic fibrosis sweat gland. Nat Genet. 1992;1:321-7. doi: 10.1038/ng0892-321.

Keown K, Brown R, Doherty DF, Houston C, McKelvey MC, Creane S, Linden D, McAuley DF, Kidney JC, Weldon S, Downey DG, Taggart CC. Airway inflammation and host responses in the era of CFTR modulators. Int J Mol Sci. 2020;21:6379. doi: 10.3390/ijms21176379.

Kerem B, Rommens JM, Buchanan JA, Markiewicz D, Cox TK, Chakravarti A, Buchwald M, Tsui LC. Identification of the cystic fibrosis gene: genetic analysis. Science. 1989; 245:1073-80. doi: 10.1126/science.2570460.

Khanolkar RA, Clark ST, Wang PW, Hwang DM, Yau YCW, Waters VJ, Guttman DS. Ecological succession of polymicrobial communities in the cystic fibrosis airways. mSystems. 2020;5:e00809-20. doi: 10.1128/mSystems.00809-20.

Kidd JF, Ramjeesingh M, Stratford F, Huan L-J, Bear CE. A heteromeric complex of the two nucleotide binding domains of cystic fibrosis transmembrane conductance regulator (CFTR) mediates ATPase activity. J Biol Chem 2004;279:41664-41669. doi: 10.1074/jbc.M407666200.

Kim Y, Jun I, Shin DH, Yoon JG, Piao H, Jung J, Park HW, Cheng MH, Bahar I, Whitcomb DC, Lee MG. Regulation of CFTR bicarbonate channel activity by WNK1: implications for pancreatitis and CFTR-related disorders. Cell Mol Gastroenterol Hepatol 2020;9:79-103. doi: 10.1016/j.jcmgh.2019.09.003.

Konstan MW, Berger M. Current understanding of the inflammatory process in cystic fibrosis: onset and etiology. Pediatr Pulmonol. 1997;24:137-42; doi: 10.1002/(sici)1099-0496(199708)24:2<137::aid-ppul13>3.0.co;2-3.

Kreda SM, Mall M, Mengos A, Rochelle L, Yankaskas J, Riordan JR, Boucher RC. Characterization of wild-type and deltaF508 cystic fibrosis transmembrane regulator in human respiratory epithelia. Mol Biol Cell. 2005;16: 2154-67. doi: 10.1091/mbc.e04-11-1010.

Krenková P, Piskácková T, Holubová A, Balašcaková M, Krulišová V, Camajová J, Turnovec M, Libik M, Norambuena P, Štambergová A, Dvoráková L, Skalická V, Bartošová J, Kucerová T, Fila L, Zemková D, Vávrová V, Koudová M, Macek M, Krebsová A, Macek M Jr. Distribution of CFTR mutations in the Czech population: positive impact of integrated clinical and laboratory expertise, detection of novel/de novo alleles and relevance for related/derived populations. J Cyst Fibros. 2013;12:532-7. doi: 10.1016/j.jcf.2012.12.002.

Kunzelmann K, Schreiber R, Hadorn HB. Bicarbonate in cystic fibrosis. J Cyst Fibros. 2017;16:653-62. doi: 10. 1016/j.jcf.2017.06.005.

Lavi E, Gileles-Hillel A, Zangen D. Somatic growth in cystic fibrosis. Curr Opin Endocrinol Diabetes Obes. 2020;27:38-46. doi: 10.1097/MED.0000000000000522.

Lewis HA, Buchanan SG, Burley SK, Conners K, Dickey M, Dorwart M, Fowler R, Gao X, Guggino WB, Hendrickson WA, Hunt JF, Kearins MC, Lorimer D, Maloney PC, Post KW, Rajashankar KR, Rutter ME, Sauder JM, Shriver S, Thibodeau PH, Thomas PJ, Zhang M, Zhao X, Emtage S. Structure of nucleotide-binding domain 1 of the cystic fibrosis transmembrane conductance regulator. EMBO J. 2004;23:282-93. doi: 10.1038/sj.emboj. 7600040.

Lewis HA, Wang C, Zhao X, Hamuro Y, Conners K, Kearins MC, Lu F, Sauder JM, Molnar KS, Coales SJ, Maloney PC, Guggino WB, Wetmore DR, Weber PC, Hunt JF. Structure and dynamics of NBD1 from CFTR characterized using crystallography and hydrogen/deuterium exchange mass spectrometry. J Mol Biol. 2010; 396:406-30. doi: 10.1016/j.jmb.2009.11.051.

Li C, Ramjeesingh M, Wang W, Garami E, Hewryk M, Lee D, Rommens JM, Galley K, Bear CE. ATPase activity of the cystic fibrosis transmembrane conductance regulator. J Biol Chem. 1996;271:28463-8. doi: 10.1074/jbc. 271.45.28463.

Li C, Naren AP. CFTR chloride channel in the apical compartments: spatiotemporal coupling to its interacting partners. Integr Biol. 2010;2:161-77. doi: 10.1039/ b924455g.

Li H, Sheppard DN. Therapeutic potential of cystic fibrosis transmembrane conductance regulator (CFTR) inhibitors in polycystic kidney disease. BioDrugs 2009; 23:203-216. doi: 10.2165/11313570-000000000-00000.

Li M-S, Cowley EA, El Hiani Y, Linsdell P. Functional organization of cytoplasmic portals controlling access to the cystic fibrosis transmembrane conductance regulator (CFTR) chloride channel pore. J Biol Chem 2018; 293:5649-5658. doi: 10.1074/jbc.RA117.001373.

Linsdell P, Tabcharani JA, Hanrahan JW. Multi-Ion mechanism for ion permeation and block in the cystic fibrosis transmembrane conductance regulator chloride channel. J Gen Physiol. 1997;110:365-77. doi: 10.1085/ jgp.110.4.365.

Linsdell P, Hanrahan JW. Adenosine triphosphate–dependent asymmetry of anion permeation in the cystic fibrosis transmembrane conductance regulator chloride channel. J Gen Physiol 1998;111:601-614. doi: 10.1085/ jgp.111.4.601.

Linsdell P. Architecture and functional properties of the CFTR channel pore. Cell Mol Life Sci 2017;74:67-83. doi: 10.1007/s00018-016-2389-5.

Liu F, Zhang Z, Csanády L, Gadsby DC, Chen J. Molecular structure of the human CFTR ion channel. Cell 2017; 169:85-95.e88. doi: 10.1007/s00018-016-2389-5.

Liu F, Zhang Z, Levit A, Levring J, Touhara KK, Shoichet BK, Chen J. Structural identification of a hotspot on CFTR for potentiation. Science. 2019;364:1184-1188. doi: 10.1126/science.aaw7611.

Luan X, Le Y, Jagadeeshan S, Murray B, Carmalt JL, Duke T, Beazley S, Fujiyama M, Swekla K, Gray B, Burmester M, Campanucci VA, Shipley A, Machen TE, Tam JS, Ianowski JP. cAMP triggers Na^+ absorption by distal airway surface epithelium in cystic fibrosis swine. Cell reports. 2021;37:109795. doi: 10.1016/j.celrep.2021. 109795.

Lukacs GL, Verkman AS. CFTR: folding, misfolding and correcting the ΔF508 conformational defect. Trends Mol Med. 2012;18:81-91. doi: 10.1016/j.molmed.2011.10. 003.

MacDonald KD1, McKenzie KR, Zeitlin PL. Cystic fibrosis transmembrane regulator protein mutations: 'class' opportunity for novel drug innovation. Paediatr Drugs. 2007;9:1-10. doi: 10.2165/00148581-200709010-00001.

Mall M, Kreda SM, Mengos A, Jensen TJ, Hirtz S, Seydewitz HH, Yankaskas J, Kunzelmann K, Riordan JR, Boucher RC. The DeltaF508 mutation results in loss of CFTR function and mature protein in native human colon. Gastroenterology. 2004;126:32-41. doi: 10.1053/j.gastro. 2003.10.049.

Mall M, Grubb BR, Harkema JR, O'Neal WK, Boucher RC. Increased airway epithelial Na^+ absorption produces cystic fibrosis-like lung disease in mice. Nat Med. 2004; 10:487-93. doi: 10.1038/nm1028.

Matsui H, Grubb BR, Tarran R, Randell SH, Gatzy JT, Davis CW, Boucher RC. Evidence for periciliary liquid layer depletion, not abnormal ion composition, in the pathogenesis of cystic fibrosis airways disease. Cell. 1998; 95:1005-15. doi: 10.1016/s0092-8674(00)81724-9.

Mickle JE, Macek M Jr, Fulmer-Smentek SB, Egan MM, Schwiebert E, Guggino W, Moss R, Cutting GR. A mutation in the cystic fibrosis transmembrane conductance regulator gene associated with elevated sweat chloride concentrations in the absence of cystic fibrosis. Hum Mol Genet. 1998;7:729-35. doi: 10.1093/hmg/7.4.729.

Montoro DT, Haber AL, Biton M, Vinarsky V, Lin B, Birket SE, Yuan F, Chen S, Leung HM, Villoria J, Rogel N, Burgin G, Tsankov AM, Waghray A, Slyper M, Waldman J, Nguyen L, Dionne D, Rozenblatt-Rosen O, Tata PR, Mou H, Shivaraju M, Bihler H, Mense M, Tearney GJ, Rowe SM, Engelhardt JF, Regev A, Rajagopal J. A revised airway epithelial hierarchy includes CFTR-expressing ionocytes. Nature. 2018;560:319-324. doi: 10.1038/s41586-018-0393-7.

Mornon JP, Lehn P, Callebaut I. Atomic model of human cystic fibrosis transmembrane conductance regulator: membrane-spanning domains and coupling interfaces. Cell Mol Life Sci. 2008;65:2594-612. doi: 10.1007/s00018-008-8249-1.

Morris-Rosendahl DJ, Edwards M, McDonnell MJ, John S, Alton EWFW, Davies JC, Simmonds NJ. Whole-gene sequencing of CFTR reveals a high prevalence of the intronic variant c.3874-4522A>G in cystic fibrosis. Am J Respir Crit Care Med. 2020; 201:1438-1441. doi: 10.1164/rccm.201908-1541LE.

Nissim-Rafinia M, Kerem B. Splicing modulation as a modifier of the CFTR function. Prog Mol Subcell Biol. 2006;44:233-54. doi: 10.1007/978-3-540-34449-0_10.

Ostedgaard LS, Meyerholz DK, Chen JH, Pezzulo AA, Karp PH, RokhlinaT, Ernst SE, Hanfland RA, Reznikov LR, Ludwig PS, Rogan MP, Davis GJ, Dohrn CL, Wohlford-Lenane C, Taft PJ, Rector MV, Hornick E, Nassar BS, Samuel M, Zhang Y, Richter SS, Uc A, Shilyansky J, Prather RS, McCray PB, Jr, Zabner J, Welsh MJ, Stoltz DA. The ΔF508 mutation causes CFTR misprocessing and cystic fibrosis-like disease in pigs. Sci Transl Med. 2011;3:74ra24. doi: 10.1126/scitranslmed.3001868.

Penque D, Mendes F, Beck S, Farinha C, Pacheco P, Nogueira P, Lavinha J, Malhó R, Amaral MD. Cystic fibrosis F508del patients have apically localized CFTR in a reduced number of airway cells. Lab Invest. 2000;80:857-68. doi: 10.1038/labinvest.3780090.

Pereira SV, Ribeiro JD, Ribeiro AF, Bertuzzo CS, Marson FAL. Novel, rare and common pathogenic variants in the *CFTR* gene screened by high-throughput sequencing technology and predicted by in silico tools. Sci Rep. 2019;9:6234. doi: 10.1038/s41598-019-42404-6.

Pérez MM, Luna MC, Pivetta OH, Keyeux G. *CFTR* gene analysis in Latin American CF patients: heterogeneous origin and distribution of mutations across the continent. J Cyst Fibros. 2007;6:194-208. doi: 10.1016/j.jcf.2006.07.004.

Pezzulo AA, Tang XX, Hoegger MJ, Alaiwa MH, Ramachandran S, Moninger TO, Karp PH, Wohlford-Lenane CL, Haagsman HP, van Eijk M, Banfi B, Horswill AR, Stoltz DA, McCray PB, Jr., Welsh MJ, Zabner J. Reduced airway surface pH impairs bacterial killing in the porcine cystic fibrosis lung. Nature 2012;487:109-113. doi:10.1038/nature11130.

Plasschaert LW, Zilionis R, Choo-Wing R, Savova V, Knehr J, Roma G, Klein AM, Jaffe AB. A single-cell atlas of the airway epithelium reveals the CFTR-rich pulmonary ionocyte. Nature. 2018;560:377-381. doi: 10.1038/s41586-018-0394-6.

Poore TS, Taylor-Cousar JL, Zemanick ET. Cardiovascular complications in cystic fibrosis: a review of the literature. J Cyst Fibros. 2022;21:18-25. doi: 10.1016/j.jcf.2021.04.016

Poulsen JH, Fischer H, Illek B, Machen TE. Bicarbonate conductance and pH regulatory capability of cystic fibrosis transmembrane conductance regulator. Proc Natl Acad Sci U. S. A 1994;91:5340-5344. doi: 10.1073/pnas.91.12.5340.

Raynal C, Corvol H. Variant classifications, databases and genotype-phenotype correlations. Arch Pediatr. 2020;27 Suppl 1:eS13-eS18. doi: 10.1016/S0929-693X(20)30045-2.

Reznikov LR. Cystic fibrosis and the nervous system. Chest. 2017;151:1147-55. doi: 10.1016/j.chest.2016.11.009.

Rich DP, Gregory RJ, Anderson MP, Manavalan P, Smith AE, Welsh MJ. Effect of deleting the R domain on CFTR-generated chloride channels. Science 1991;253:205-207. doi: 10.1126/science.1712985.

Rich DP, Berger HA, Cheng SH, Travis SM, Saxena M, Smith AE, Welsh MJ. Regulation of the cystic fibrosis transmembrane conductance regulator Cl^- channel by negative charge in the R domain. J Biol Chem. 1993;268:20259-67.

Riordan JR. CFTR function and prospects for therapy. Annu Rev Biochem. 2008;77:701-26. doi: 10.1146/annurev.biochem.75.103004.142532.

Riordan JR, Rommens JM, Kerem B, Alon N, Rozmahel R, Grzelczak Z, Zielenski J, Lok S, Plavsic N, Chou JL, Drumm ML, Iannuzzi MC,Collins FS, Tsui L-C. Identification of the cystic fibrosis gene: cloning and characterization of complementary DNA. Science. 1989; 245:1066-73. doi: 10.1126/science.2475911.

Roesch EA, Nichols DP, Chmiel, JF. Inflammation in cystic fibrosis: an update. Pediatr Pulmonol. 2018;53:S30-50. doi: 10.1002/ppul.24129.

Sagel SD, Chmiel JF, Konstan MW. Sputum biomarkers of inflammation in cystic fibrosis lung disease. Proc Am Thorac Soc. 2007;4:406-17. doi:10.1513/pats.200703-044BR.

Saint-Criq V, Gray MA. Role of CFTR in epithelial physiology. Cell Mol Life Sci 2017;74:93-115. doi: 10.1007/s00018-016-2391-y.

Sathe M, Sharma PB, Savant AP. Year in review 2020: nutrition and gastrointestinal disease in cystic fibrosis. Pediatr Pulmonol. 2021;56:3120-5. doi: 10.1002/ppul.25587.

Scholl D, Sigoillot M, Overtus M, Martinez RC, Martens C, Wang Y, Pardon E, Laeremans T, Garcia-Pino A, Steyaert J, Sheppard DN, Hendrix J, Govaerts C. A topological switch in CFTR modulates channel activity and sensitivity to unfolding. Nat Chem Biol 2021;17:989-997. doi: 10.1038/s41589-021-00844-0.2021.

Schwiebert EM, Benos DJ, Egan ME, Stutts MJ, Guggino WB. CFTR Is a conductance regulator as well as a chloride channel. Physiol Rev. 1999;79 (1 Suppl):S145-66. doi: 10.1152/physrev.1999.79.1.S145.

Sermet-Gaudelus I, Vallée B, Urbin I, Torossi T, Marianovski R, Fajac A, Feuillet MN, Bresson JL, Lenoir G, Bernaudin JF, Edelman A. Normal function of the cystic fibrosis conductance regulator protein can be associated with homozygous (Delta)F508 mutation. Pediatr Res. 2002;52:628-35. doi: 10.1203/00006450-200211000-00005.

Serohijos AWR, Hegedus T, Aleksandrov AA, He L, Cui L, Dokholyan NV, Riordan JR. Phenylalanine-508 mediates a cytoplasmic-membrane domain contact in the CFTR 3D structure crucial to assembly and channel function. Proc Natl Acad Sci U. S. A. 2008;105:3256-3261. doi: 10.1073/pnas.0800254105.

Shah VS, Chivukula RR, Lin B, Waghray A, Rajagopal J. Cystic Fibrosis and the cells of the airway epithelium: What are ionocytes and what do they do? Annu Rev Pathol. 2022;17:23-46. doi: 10.1146/annurev-pathol-042420-094031.

Sheppard DN, Rich DP, Ostedgaard LS, Gregory RJ, Smith AE, Welsh MJ. Mutations in CFTR associated with mild-disease-form Cl^- channels with altered pore properties. Nature 1993;362:160-164. doi: 10.1038/362160a0.

Shteinberg M, Haq IJ, Polineni D, Davies JC. Cystic fibrosis. Lancet. 2021a;397:2195-211. doi: 10.1016/S0140-6736(20)32542-3.

Shteinberg M, Taylor-Cousar JL, Durieu I, Cohen-Cymberknoh M. Fertility and pregnancy in cystic fibrosis. Chest. 2021b. DOI: 10.1016/j.chest.2021.07.024

Smith SS, Steinle ED, Meyerhoff ME, Dawson DC. Cystic fibrosis transmembrane conductance regulator. Physical basis for lyotropic anion selectivity patterns. J Gen Physiol 1999;114:799-818. doi: 10.1085/jgp.114.6.799.

Sosnay PR, Siklosi KR, Van Goor F, Kaniecki K, Yu H, Sharma N, Ramalho AS, Amaral MD, Dorfman R, Zielenski J, Masica DL, Karchin R, Millen L, Thomas PJ, Patrinos GP, Corey M, Lewis MH, Rommens JM, Castellani C, Penland CM, Cutting GR. Defining the disease liability of variants in the cystic fibrosis transmembrane conductance regulator gene. Nat Genet. 2013;45:1160-7. doi: 10.1038/ng.2745.

Stanke F, Ballmann M, Bronsveld I, Dörk T, Gallati S, Laabs U, Derichs N, Ritzka M, Posselt HG, Harms HK, Griese M, Blau H, Mastella G, Bijman J, Veeze H, Tümmler B. Diversity of the basic defect of homozygous *CFTR* mutation genotypes in humans. J Med Genet. 2008;45:47-54. doi: 10.1136/jmg.2007.053561.

Stanke F, Pallenberg S, Tamm S, Hedtfeld S, Eichhorn EM, Minso R, Sauer-Heilborn A, Ringshausen FC, Junge S, Welte T, Hansen G, Tümmler B, Dittrich AM. Changes in intestinal CFTR protein expression in p.Phe508del homozygous and compound heterozygous patients with cystic fibrosis prior and during elexacaftor / tezacaftor / ivacaftor therapy. submitted 2022.

Stoltz DA, Meyerholz DK, Welsh MJ. Origins of cystic fibrosis lung disease. N Engl J Med. 2015; 372: 351-62. doi: 10.1056/NEJMra1300109.

Stutts MJ, Canessa CM, Olsen JC, Hamrick M, Cohn JA, Rossier BC, Boucher RC. CFTR as a cAMP-dependent regulator of sodium channels. Science 1995;269:847-850. doi: 10.1126/science.7543698.

Szollosi A, Muallem DR, Csanády L, Vergani P. Mutant cycles at CFTR's non-canonical ATP-binding site support little interface separation during gating. J Gen Physiol 2011;137:549-562. doi: 10.1085/jgp.201110608.

Tang L, Fatehi M, Linsdell P. Mechanism of direct bicarbonate transport by the CFTR anion channel. J Cyst Fibros. 2009;8:115-21. doi: 10.1016/j.jcf.2008.10.004.

Thibodeau PH, Richardson JM 3rd, Wang W, Millen L, Watson J, Mendoza JL, Du K, Fischman S, Senderowitz H, Lukacs GL, Kirk K, Thomas PJ. The cystic fibrosis-causing mutation deltaF508 affects multiple steps in cystic fibrosis transmembrane conductance regulator biogenesis. J Biol Chem. 2010;285:35825-35. doi: 10.1074/jbc.M110.131623.

Tsai MF, Li M, Hwang TC. Stable ATP binding mediated by a partial NBD dimer of the CFTR chloride channel. J Gen Physiol. 2010;135:399-414. doi: 10.1085/jgp.201010399.

van Barneveld A, Stanke F, Tamm S, Siebert B, Brandes G, Derichs N, Ballmann M, Junge S, Tümmler B. Functional analysis of F508del CFTR in native human colon. Biochim Biophys Acta. 2010;1802:1062-9. doi: 10.1016/j.bbadis.2010.08.001.

Van Goor F, Yu H, Burton B, Hoffman BJ. Effect of ivacaftor on CFTR forms with missense mutations associated with defects in protein processing or function. J Cyst Fibros. 2014;13:29-36. doi: 10.1016/j.jcf.2013.06.008.

Veit G, Avramescu RG, Chiang AN, Houck SA, Cai Z, Peters KW, Hong JS, Pollard HB, Guggino WB, Balch WE, Skach WR, Cutting GR, Frizzell RA, Sheppard DN, Cyr DM, Sorscher EJ, Brodsky JL, Lukacs GL. From CFTR biology toward combinatorial pharmacotherapy: expanded classification of cystic fibrosis mutations. Mol Biol Cell 2016;27:424-433. doi: 10.1091/mbc.E14-04-0935.

Vergani P, Lockless SW, Nairn AC, Gadsby DC. CFTR channel opening by ATP-driven tight dimerization of its nucleotide-binding domains. Nature. 2005;433:876-80. doi: 10.1038/nature03313.

Wang X, Venable J, LaPointe P, Hutt DM, Koulov AV, Coppinger J, Gurkan C, Kellner W, Matteson J, Plutner H, Riordan JR, Kelly JW, Yates JR 3rd, Balch WE. Hsp90 cochaperone Aha1 downregulation rescues misfolding of CFTR in cystic fibrosis. Cell. 2006;127:803-15. doi: 10.1016/j.cell.2006.09.043.

Ward CL, Omura S, Kopito RR. Degradation of CFTR by the ubiquitin-proteasome pathway. Cell. 1995;83:121-7. doi: 10.1016/0092-8674(95)90240-6.

Watson MS1, Cutting GR, Desnick RJ, Driscoll DA, Klinger K, Mennuti M, Palomaki GE, Popovich BW, Pratt VM, Rohlfs EM, Strom CM, Richards CS, Witt DR, Grody WW. Cystic fibrosis population carrier screening: 2004 revision of American College of Medical Genetics mutation panel. Genet Med. 2004;6:387-91. doi: 10. 1097/01.gim.0000139506.11694.7c.

Webster MJ, Tarran R. Slippery when wet: airway surface liquid homeostasis and mucus hydration. Curr Top Membr. 2018;81:293-335. doi: 10.1016/bs.ctm.2018.08. 004.

Welsh MJ, Smith AE. Molecular mechanisms of CFTR chloride channel dysfunction in cystic fibrosis. Cell. 1993;73:1251-4. doi: 10.1016/0092-8674(93)90353-r.

Will K, Dörk T, Stuhrmann M, Meitinger T, Bertele-Harms R, Tümmler B, Schmidtke J. A novel exon in the cystic fibrosis transmembrane conductance regulator gene activated by the nonsense mutation E92X in airway epithelial cells of patients with cystic fibrosis. J Clin Invest. 1994;93:1852-9. doi: 10.1172/JCI117172.

Will K, Dörk T, Stuhrmann M, von der Hardt H, Ellemunter H, Tümmler B, Schmidtke J. Transcript analysis of CFTR nonsense mutations in lymphocytes and nasal epithelial cells from cystic fibrosis patients. Hum Mutat. 1995;5:210-20. doi: 10.1002/humu.1380050305.

Winter MC, Welsh MJ. Stimulation of CFTR activity by its phosphorylated R domain. Nature. 1997;389:294-6. doi: 10.1038/38514.

World Health Organization. WHO report 2004. http://www.who.int/genomics/publications/en/

Zajac M, Dreano E, Edwards A, Planelles G, Sermet-Gaudelus I. Airway surface liquid pH regulation in airway epithelium current understandings and gaps in knowledge. Int J Mol Sci. 2021;22:3384. doi: 10.3390/ijms22073384.

Zhang W, Zhang Z, Zhang Y, Naren AP. CFTR-NHERF2-LPA_2 complex in the airway and gut epithelia. Int J Mol Sci. 2017;18:1896. doi: 10.3390/ijms18091896.

Zhang Z, Chen J. Atomic structure of the cystic fibrosis transmembrane conductance regulator. Cell 2016;167: 1586-1597.e1589. doi: 10.1016/j.cell.2016.11.014.

Zhang Z, Liu F, Chen J. Conformational changes of CFTR upon phosphorylation and ATP Binding. Cell. 2017;170:483-491.e8. doi: 10.1016/j.cell.2017.06.041.

Zhang Z, Liu F, Chen J. Molecular structure of the ATP-bound, phosphorylated human CFTR. Proc Natl Acad Sci U. S. A. 2018;115:12757-12762. doi: 10.1073/pnas. 1815287115.

Ziêtkiewicz E, Rutkiewicz E, Pogorzelski A, Klimek B, Voelkel K, Witt M. CFTR mutations spectrum and the efficiency of molecular diagnostics in Polish cystic fibrosis patients. PLoS One. 2014;9:e89094. doi: 10.1371/journal.pone.0089094.

2. Bioassays to assess CFTR function in humans

2.1. Sweat chloride test and β-adrenergic sweat secretion

Tanja Gonska

The dramatic change of the sweat chloride concentration that was observed in cystic fibrosis patients carrying p.Gly551Asp mutations following treatment with the first approved CFTR-targeting drug, ivacaftor, has highlighted the role of the sweat chloride test as a biomarker test in CF (Accurso et al., 2010; Ramsey et al., 2011). This immediate drug effect on the sweat chloride concentration confirmed causality between the basic CFTR defect and the pathophysiological observation of chloride impermeability in sweat ducts of CF patients, which was described prior to the identification of the *CFTR* gene (Quinton, 1983).

The quantitative pilocarpine iontophoresis test (QPIT) was established by Gibson and Cooke (1959) and has since served as the standard diagnostic test in establishing or excluding a diagnosis of Cystic Fibrosis worldwide. It is an integral part of the North American and European CF diagnostic guidelines (Farrell et al., 2008; de Boeck et al., 2006). Further, it has been implemented in all CF centres taking part in CF newborn screening programs as a confirmatory diagnostic test for CF (Farrell et al., 2008). It is now also integral part as outcome parameter in clinical trials to test the efficacy of CFTR modulators as well as used to provide proof of clinical modulator effectiveness for drug funding agencies at an individual patient level (Accurso et al., 2014; Fidler et al., 2017; Middleton et al., 2019).

This test is based on the 3 steps procedure of

a) sweat stimulation by iontophoresis using pilocarpine as a cholinergic agent,

b) sweat collection with a gauze patch or a collector tubing system (Macroduct®) and

c) biochemical analysis of the chloride concentration in the sweat (Gibson and Cooke, 1959; Green and Kirk, 2007). The reference ranges for the QPIT were originally established in patients presenting with severe CF disease symptoms on one hand and a mixed group of healthy controls and patients presenting only with lung disease or gastrointestinal symptoms on the other hand (Gibson and Cooke, 1959).

Today we recognize CF as a disease spectrum comprising a range of different CF phenotypes, which is paralleled by the number and severity of the *CFTR* mutations (☞ Figure 2.1). Broadening the disease spectrum has revealed the diagnostic limitations of the sweat chloride test as there are large overlaps in sweat chloride concentration between patients with no disease symptoms and *CFTR* mutations, patients with disease symptoms and *CFTR* mutations of unknown clinical significance as well as patients with disease symptoms and two CF causing mutations (Durno et al., 2002; Wilschanski et al., 2006; Gonska et al., 2012).

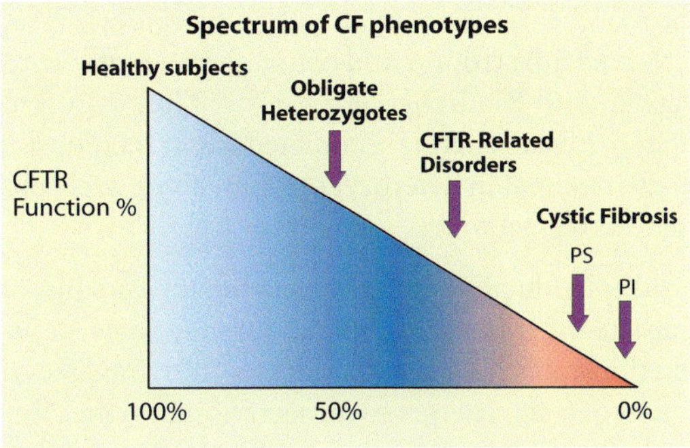

Figure 2.1: Current model of the spectrum of CF phenotypes. PS = pancreatic sufficient; PI = pancreatic insufficient.

Adjunctive tests assessing CFTR function in other epithelial tissues such as nasal mucosa (nasal potential difference) and intestinal tissue (intestinal current measurements) have been implemented in a few specialized CF centres to close this diagnostic gap. However, an argument can be made that the sweat gland offers better features for new diagnostic test development, since sweat glands:

1) highly express CFTR,

2) are not altered by secondary inflammatory changes and

3) are easily accessible for testing (Quinton, 2007).

While the currently used QPIT sweat test measures CFTR in its absorptive function at the level of the sweat duct, CFTR is also expressed in the sweat se-

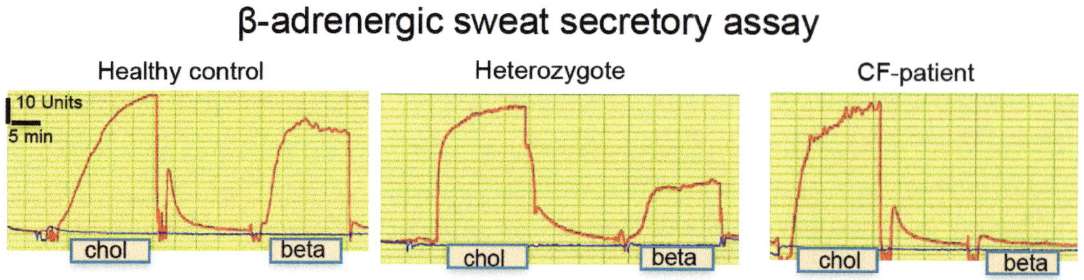

Figure 2.2: Examples of the original tracing measuring sweat secretion with an evaporimeter (Cyber Derm, Broomall, PA) following a) sweat stimulation with a cholinergic agent (chol), b) inhibition of the cholinergic sweating with atropine and c) sweat stimulation with a β-adrenergic cocktail (isoproterenol, aminophylline and atropine, beta). Whereas the cholinergic sweat secretion varies among individuals, the β-adrenergic sweat secretion is 50% in heterozygous subjects compared to healthy controls and completely absent in patients with CF.

cretory coil where it functions as a chloride secretory channel. In the early 1980s Sato and Sato (1984) as well as Behm et al. (1987) made the discovery that CFTR-mediated sweat secretion can be detected in individual subjects following inhibition of the thermoregulative, cholinergic sweat secretion with atropine and consequent sweat stimulation with β-adrenergic agonists. They reported that the β-adrenergic stimulated sweat secretion is half-maximal in heterozygotes and completely absent in CF patients.

The introduction of an evaporimeter capable of measuring this low volume β-adrenergic sweat secretion rates has recently allowed moving assessment of β-adrenergic sweat secretion into the clinical setting (Quinton et al., 2012; Salinas et al., 2020). The test protocol follows the principle of the original experiments

1) pilocarpine for cholinergic sweat stimulation,

2) atropine for inhibition of cholinergic sweat stimulation and

3) a beta-cocktail of isoproterenol, aminophylline and atropine for β-adrenergic sweat stimulation. The sweat gland secretory responses to this stimulation sequence can be recorded by placing the evaporimeter probe on the stimulated skin area. Mineral oil is applied before the measurement to avoid interference of transdermal transpiration. Following this protocol, the β-adrenergic sweat secretory test is the first biomarker assay indicating half-maximal CFTR function in heterozygous subjects carrying one *CFTR* mutation. It also identifies all CF patients including those carrying *CFTR* mutations that are associated with normal or borderline sweat chloride concentrations, e.g. 3849+10kbC>T and p.Asp1152His (☞ Figure 2.2). Next to the use of an evaporimeter Jeff Wine and his group have developed a method that allows assessing the β-adrenergic stimulated sweat rate on an individual sweat gland basis using the "bubble method" (Kim et al., 2016). Using this method sweat stimulation is the same as described above but sweat rate assessment is performed by following the growth of single droplets under a microscope. CFTR modulator effects on the β-adrenergic sweat secretion rate have been described with this "bubble method" (Char et al., 2017; Kim et al., 2018; Pallenberg et al., 2021). Meanwhile novel standardized protocols of stimulation procedure, automatic image processing and data quality control are available (Bergamini et al., 2018; Treggiari et al., 2021; Pallenberg et al., 2021). Images of sweat bubble formation are recorded by a USB-microscope camera every 2 seconds and the sweat rate in nl/min is calculated from the kinetics of the median sweat bubble size over time (Pallenberg et al., 2021). Since the β-adrenergic sweat secretory test provides additional information about CFTR function, it may thus be used as an adjunctive diagnostic tool in uncertain diagnostic cases (☞ Figure 2.3).

In summary, the sweat gland serves as an easy assessable organ for testing CFTR function either measuring CFTR function in its absorptive role at the level of the sweat duct or in its secretory role at the level of the sweat secretory coil.

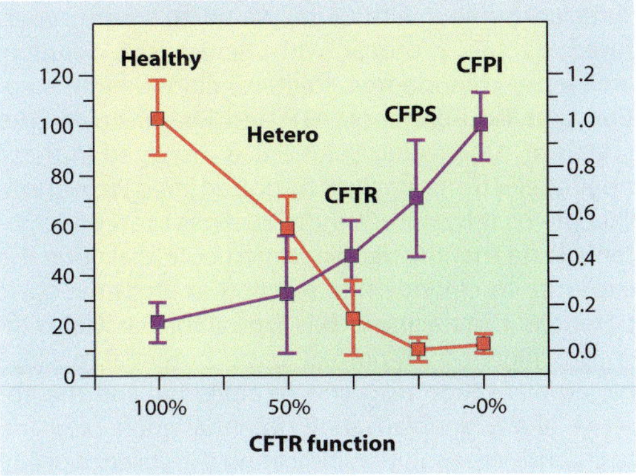

Figure 2.3: Spectrum of CFTR function represented by sweat [Cl⁻] and β-adrenergic sweat secretory test. The QPIT (lilac, left scale) and β-adrenergic sweat secretory tests (red, right scale) were done in parallel in the same subjects belonging to one of the following categories: healthy controls (Healthy), heterozygote (Hetero), CFTR-related disorder (CFTR), pancreatic sufficient (CFPS) and pancreatic insufficient CF (CFPI) patients. While the QPIT distinguished between CFPS and CFPI patients, the β-adrenergic sweat secretory test discriminated between Healthy, Hetero, CFTR-related and CF (modified from Quinton P et al., β-adrenergic sweat secretion as a diagnostic test for cystic fibrosis. Am J Respir Crit Care Med 2012;186:732-9).

2.2. Nasal transepithelial potential difference measurements

Sophia Theres Pallenberg and Burkhard Tümmler

2.2.1. Background

The basic defect in cystic fibrosis (CF) translates into an impaired permeability of the apical epithelial membrane for chloride and bicarbonate. In the early 1980s Michael Knowles and colleagues discovered that the impaired chloride conductance can be directly measured in the nasal respiratory epithelium *in vivo* (Knowles et al., 1981; 1983a; 1983b). Although it was evident from the very beginning that the anomalous nasal transepithelial electric potential difference (NPD) could be exploited to make the diagnosis of CF, its application to daily clinical practise remained restricted to a few dedicated CF clinics, because the measurement of the NPD required manual skills and expertise and the validity and reproducibility of individual recordings were jeopardized by relatively low signal-to-noise ratios.

Unreliability, excessive artifacts, and lack of standardization of the testing systems were gradually overcome by the publication of protocols (Middleton et al., 1994; Knowles et al., 1995), the introduction of standard operating procedures (SOPs; Standaert et al., 2004) and the randomized multicenter comparison of NPD techniques (Solomon et al., 2010). A quantum leap was achieved by the introduction of electronic data capture that was accompanied by the publication of detailed and easy-to-follow SOPs by the CFFT Therapeutics Development Network Coordinating Center (2009) and the European Cystic Fibrosis Society (ECFS) Diagnostic Network Working Group & Clinical Trials Network (2013). Hence, NPD has become an established biomarker in the diagnostic setting (Minso et al., 2020) and an endpoint of clinical trials of CFTR modulators (Sermet-Gaudelus et al., 2021).

2.2.2. Principle of the assay

NPD measures the transepithelial nasal potential difference between the nasal respiratory epithelium and the subcutaneous space in the forearm. The electric potential of the nasal floor is explored with an agar-filled catheter at its most electronegative position and is continuously recorded with two calomel or Ag/AgCl electrodes. The basic electric potential during superfusion with a buffered salt solution is more negative in individuals with CF than in non-CF controls (☞ Figure 2.4a-c). Subsequent superfusion with an amiloride-containing salt solution blocks the sodium conductance, which is mediated by the epithelial sodium channel ENaC. The amiloride blockage of ENaC induces a hyperpolarization potential that is higher in CF than non-CF. Next, the switch to superfusion with a buffered chloride-free gluconate solution (ΔCl-free) induces a depolarization potential because the CFTR-mediated chloride conductance is blocked. Change to isoproterenol-containing chloride-free solution (Iso) will further increase the depolarization potential because more CFTR channels are activated by the β_2-sympathicomimetic agonist isoproterenol. The cumulative responses to ΔCl-free+Iso solutions are well above −10 mV in non-CF, whereas individuals with CF harbouring no functional CFTR in their upper airway epithelium show no clearly discernible depolarization signal. Exocrine pancreatic sufficient (PS) individuals with CF typically express some residual CFTR-mediated chloride conductance in the nasal respiratory epithelium, which shows up in the NPD by a small depolarization potential of a few mV. Next, the purinergic receptors are activated with ATP to induce some non-CFTR-mediated chloride conductance, which is seen in both non-CF and CF nostrils. Figure 2.4a-c shows typical tracings of a non-CF control (a), CF with two loss-of-function *CFTR* mutations (b) and CF with at least one PS *CFTR* mutation (c).

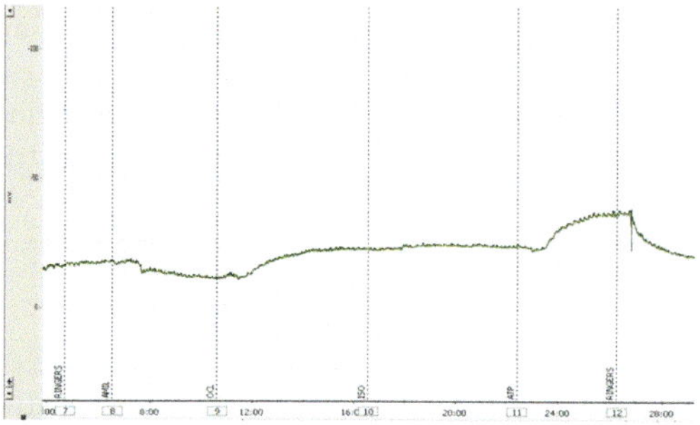

a

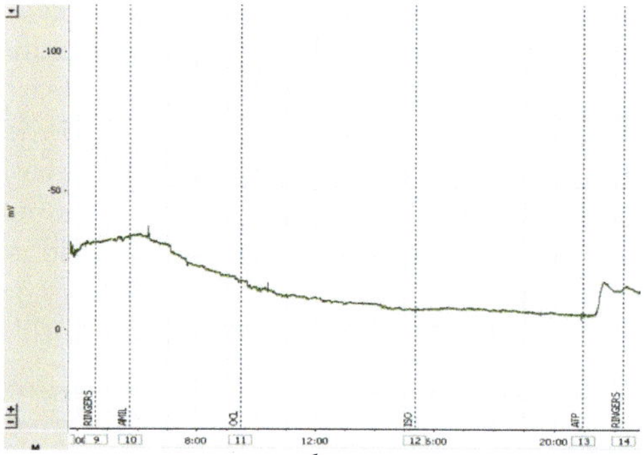

b

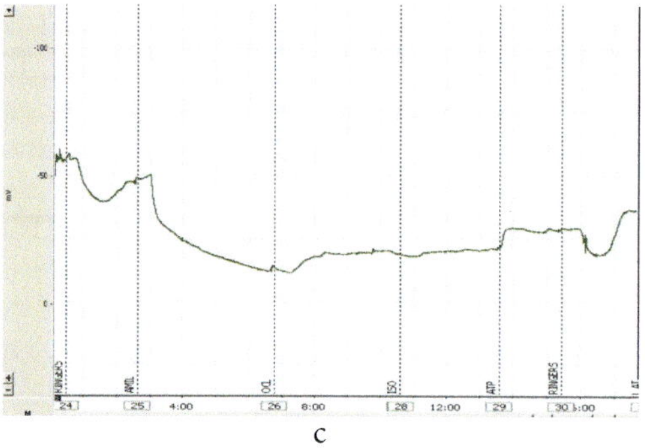

c

Figure 2.4a-c: Nasal potential difference measurements in a healthy non-CF subject (a), a F508del homozygous subject with CF (b) and an exocrine pancreas-sufficient subject with CF (c). All nostrils were superfused as per protocol with Ringer salt solution, amiloride, chloride-free solution, chloride-free solution plus isoproterenol, ATP and Ringer again. The switch of superfusing solutions is indicated in these original electronic tracings by dotted lines. Please note that the healthy non-CF individual has a low basic potential and that the depolarisation potential upon the exposure to chloride-free solution exceeds the basic potential. The tracing in **b** is typical for classical PI CF with a higher-than-normal basic potential, a large hyperpolarisation response to amiloride and the absence of any depolarisation potential upon exposure to chloride-free solution indicating the absence of any CFTR-mediated chloride conductance. The tracing in **c** was recorded at the day of diagnosis of a 36-year-old female who had been diagnosed before as suffering from non-CF bronchiectasis. CF had been suspected on numerous occasions but was excluded every time because of normal chloride concentrations in sweat tests. Please note the large negative basic potential in the CF range and the depolarisation potential in the borderline range between CF and non-CF indicating substantial residual CFTR-mediated chloride conductance in this subject. The subsequent *CFTR* mutation analysis uncovered a stop mutation and the splice mutation 3849+10 kb C-T as disease-causing *CFTR* alleles the latter being known to be associated with normal sweat test values.

2.2.3. Applications

NPD has been used as a diagnostic test for CF since the late 1980s and was accepted as a diagnostic procedure equal to sweat chloride >60 mmol/L and/or detection of two CF-causing mutations in 1998 in the Cystic Fibrosis Foundation (CFF) consensus statement (Rosenstein and Cutting, 1998). NPD is primarily applied to make a diagnosis in subjects with an intermediate or borderline sweat test. Besides the criterion of the CFTR-associated cumulative response to ΔCl-free+Iso two more discriminatory diagnostic NPD scores have been developed that evaluate both the amiloride-induced hyperpolarization and the cumulative ΔCl-free+Iso depolarization (Wilschanski et al., 2001; Sermet-Gaudelus et al., 2010). Moreover, the combination of sweat chloride and two NPD parameters (ΔCl-free+Iso and ΔAmil+Cl-free+Iso) has shown to be useful for the diagnostic determination of patients with questionable CF (Ooi et al., 2014).

NPD is a biomarker of CFTR activity in the airway epithelium. Hence, it can be utilized in clinical trials to assess the efficacy of drugs whether they can modulate the basic defect in CF. NPD has been applied as a secondary endpoint in phase 2 studies with ivacaftor (Accurso et al., 2010), lumacaftor (Clancy et al., 2012) and ataluren (Kerem et al., 2008) and in post-approval studies on combination therapy with lumacaftor/ivacaftor (Graeber et al., 2018) and elexacaftor/tezacaftor/ivacaftor (Graeber et al., 2022). In the phase 2 study the average changes of ΔCl-free+Iso upon treatment with ivacaftor in subjects with CF with at least one p.Gly551Asp mutation was determined to be –7 mV at the highest dose of 250 mg (Accurso et al., 2010). Figure 2.5a+b shows the NPD recordings of a p.Gly551Asp compound heterozygous patient from the authors' clinic. During treatment with ivacaftor the standard potential and the hyperpolarization potential decreased and the ΔCl-free+ Iso response increased from zero above the average –7 mV to a value in the gray zone between non-CF and CF. This example illustrates the potential of NPD as a measure of efficacy in the upcoming era of personalized medicine for individuals with CF.

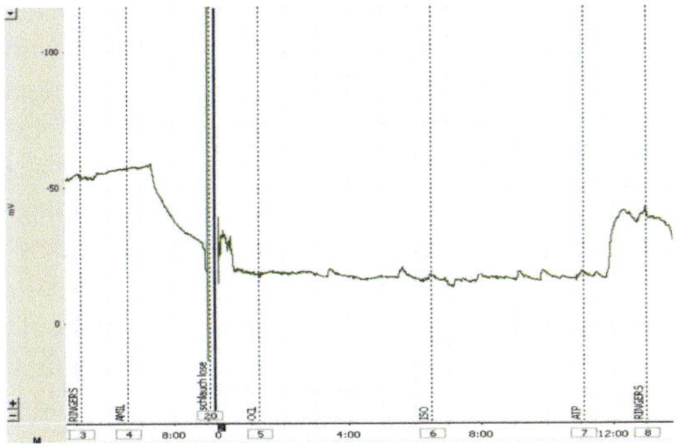

a

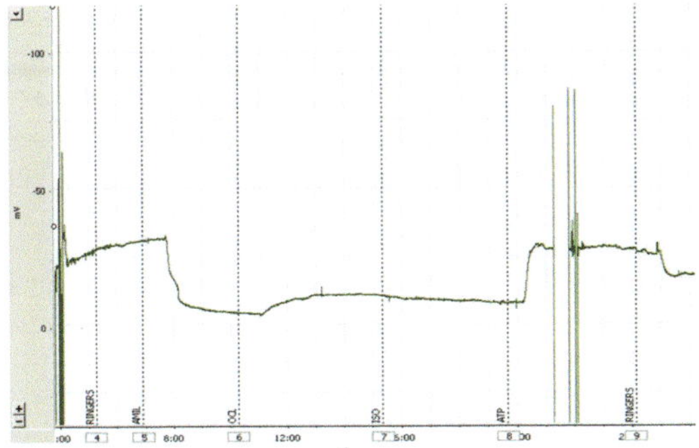

b

Figure 2.5a+b: Nasal potential difference measurements of a subject with CF who is compound heterozygous for G551D prior (**a**) and during treatment with the CFTR potentiator ivacaftor (**b**). Scales of the two tracings are the same for voltage (ordinate) and time (abscissa). With ivacaftor the basic potential and the hyperpolarisation potential decreased in the direction of the normal range. Chloride-free solution evoked a depolarisation potential in the gray zone between CF and non-CF indicating substantial CFTR-mediated chloride conductance that was absent prior to therapy with ivacaftor.

2.3. Intestinal current measurements

Simon Y. Graeber and Marcus A. Mall

2.3.1. Principle of the assay

Bioelectric measurements in rectal biopsy tissues, also known as intestinal current measurements (ICM), provide a sensitive bioassay for assessment of CFTR function *ex vivo* (Mall et al., 2004; De Jonge et al., 2004; Li et al., 2004). The technique takes advantage of relatively high levels of CFTR expression reflected by a high signal-to-noise ratio in rectal mucosa compared to the airways. ICM can be performed safely and easily at any age group including infants. Superficial biopsies of the rectal mucosa (i.e. only epithelial layer, no muscle layer) are obtained by forceps or suction biopsy and are immediately mounted in perfused or circulating small aperture Ussing chambers and equilibrated in physiological buffer solution at 37°C. After equilibration, basal bioelectric properties including transepithelial voltage (V_{te}), resistance (R_{te}) and short circuit current (I_{sc}) are recorded under open-circuit or short-circuit conditions, and effects of pharmacological stimuli on intestinal ion transport can be studied *ex vivo* in a controlled setting (Mall et al., 2004; De Jonge et al., 2004; Li et al., 2004).

The ICM technique was originally developed to study normal ion transport physiology and determine the basic CF defects in the intestine (Hardcastle et al., 1991; Veeze et al., 1991; Mall et al., 1998; 1999; 2000; Kunzelmann and Mall, 2002). These studies demonstrated that CFTR is the dominant Cl^- channel responsible for Cl^- and fluid secretion in human colon. As illustrated in Figure 2.6, stimulation of CFTR-mediated Cl^- secretion requires cAMP-dependent activation of luminal CFTR Cl^- channels and basolateral K^+ channels that hyperpolarize the membrane potential and thus provide the electrochemical driving force for luminal Cl^- exit (☞ Figure 2.6A). In contrast to the airways, rectal mucosa does not express a prominent alternative Ca^{2+}-activated Cl^- channel (CaCC). However, Ca^{2+}-dependent co-activation, e.g. by cholinergic stimulation with carbachol, activates Ca^{2+}-sensitive K^+ channels in the basolateral membrane and thereby augments the driving force for luminal Cl^- secretion via CFTR (☞ Figure 2.6A; Mall et al., 1998; 1999; 2000).

For standardized testing of CFTR function in rectal biopsies, the apical Na^+ conductance is inhibited by amiloride (10 µmol/L) and tissue synthesis of prostaglandin, an important endogenous agonist of the cAMP pathway, is blocked by the cyclooxygenase inhibitor indomethacin (10 µmol/L). Under these conditions, epithelial Na^+ channels (ENaC) as well as CFTR Cl^- channels are inactive and the transepithelial V_{te} and I_{sc} approach zero. Next, intracellular cAMP levels are elevated by adding forskolin (10 µmol/L), an activator of the adenylate cyclase (AC) in combination with the phosphodiesterase inhibitor isobutylmethylxanthin (IBMX, 100 µmol/L). In rectal tissue from healthy individuals, cAMP-dependent activation induces CFTR-mediated Cl^- secretion that is reflected by an increase in lumen-negative V_{te} and I_{sc}. This Cl^- secretory response is substantially augmented by cholinergic co-activation with carbachol (CCH, 100 µmol/l; ☞ Figure 2.6A). In patients with CF, ICM allows to discriminate between two functional phenotypes. In the larger group, ICM detects little or no functional CFTR. Instead, cAMP- and Ca^{2+}-dependent activation commonly induce inverse lumen-positive responses reflecting luminal K^+ secretion (☞ Figure 2.6B; Mall et al., 2000). CF patients with this ICM pattern typically carry two 'severe' *CFTR* mutations (class I to III) and present with a classical CF phenotype including exocrine pancreatic insufficiency (PI; Mall et al., 2004; Hirtz et al., 2004). In the second group encompassing ~15-20% of all CF patients, ICM detects residual CFTR function evidenced by an attenuated Cl^- secretory (i.e. lumen-negative) response to cAMP-dependent activation and a biphasic response to cholinergic co-activation (☞ Figure 2.6C; Hirtz et al., 2004; Veeze et al., 1994; Sousa et al., 2012). Patients with this ICM response typically carry at least one 'mild' *CFTR* mutation (class IV and V) and present with a milder or atypical form of CF including later age at diagnosis, less severe impairment of weight-for-height and lung function, and long-term pancreatic sufficiency (PS; Hirtz et al., 2004).

2.3.2. Applications

Based on these results, the ICM technique has been successfully used to elucidate the relationship between CFTR Cl^- channel function, *CFTR* genotypes and the clinical phenotype (Veeze et al., 1994; Hirtz et al., 2004; Stanke et al., 2008), as well as the role of genetic modifiers including genes that modulate the folding and trafficking of the most common mutant Phe508del-CFTR (Bronsveld et al., 2000; 2001; Stanke et al., 2014). More recently, the ICM technique has obtained attention as a diagnostic tool in the work-up of patients with an equivocal diagnosis due to borderline sweat tests, inconclusive genetic testing or atypical clinical presentation (De Boeck et al., 2013), and has been established at a number of diagnostic reference centers in Germany, the Netherlands, Israel, Portugal, Brazil and the USA for this purpose (Derichs et al., 2010; Sousa et al., 2012; Clancy et al., 2013; Minso et al., 2020; Silva et al., 2020). In contrast to nasal PD measurements that require patient cooperation, ICM can be reliably performed at any age group and is therefore, also suitable for the diagnostic work-up of infants with positive CF newborn screening and equivocal sweat test results (Sommerburg et al., 2010; Bagheri-Hanson et al., 2014). As mentioned above, detection of residual CFTR function by ICM is associated with a milder CF phenotype including long-term pancreatic sufficiency (PS). Therefore, diagnostic ICM can also have prognostic value especially in CF patients in whom the two disease-causing *CFTR* mutations have not been identified, as well as in patients carrying mutations with unknown functional consequences (Hirtz et al., 2004; Hentschel et al., 2012; Minso et al., 2020).

Finally, ICM has recently been established as a sensitive biomarker of CFTR function in response to CFTR modulator therapy. An earlier proof-of-concept study tested the *ex vivo* effects of the potentiator 1-EBIO (1-ethyl-2-benzimidazolone), a compound that augments CFTR-mediated Cl^- secretion via several mechanisms including

- direct effects on CFTR,

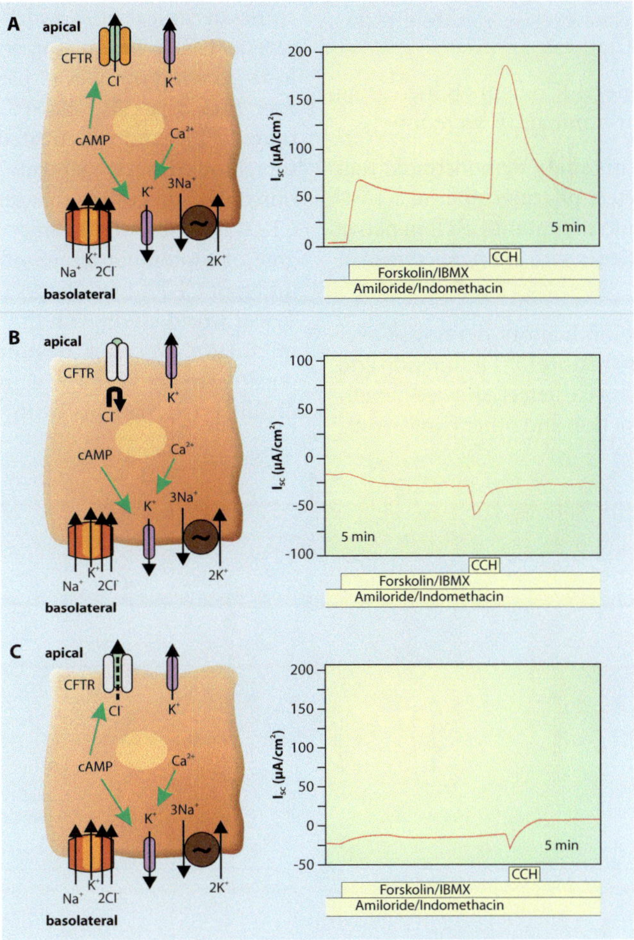

Figure 2.6: Assessment of wild-type and mutant CFTR function by intestinal current measurement (ICM). CFTR-mediated Cl^- secretion can be determined from bioelectric responses of rectal biopsies to cAMP-mediated and cholinergic activation, as illustrated in colonocyte cell models and original Ussing chamber recordings of transepithelial voltage (V_{te}) in rectal tissues from a healthy individual (**A**), a CF patient with 'severe' CFTR mutations (R1162X/Q552X) and lack of CFTR Cl^- channel function (**B**), and a CF patient with 'mild' CFTR mutations (S1159F/S1159F) expressing residual CFTR function (**C**). ICM measurements are performed in the presence of amiloride to block ENaC-mediated Na^+ absorption and indomethacin to suppress formation of prostaglandin and endogenous cAMP levels. V_{te} deflections are obtained by pulsed current injection and reflect R_{te}. **A:** Normal colonocytes are equipped with the Na^+-K^+-ATPase, K^+ channels and the Na^+-K^+-$2Cl^-$ cotransporter (NKCC1) in the basolateral membrane, which work in concert to maintain intracellular ion homeostasis, generate the membrane potential and take up Cl^- from the blood side into the cell. In the apical membrane, CFTR Cl^- channels and K^+ channels are responsible for KCl secretion. In healthy individuals, elevation of intracellular cAMP results in sustained activation of CFTR Cl^- channels and basolateral K^+ channels that provide the electrochemical driving force for luminal Cl^- secretion. Elevation of intracellular Ca^+ activates Ca^+-dependent K^+ channels that further increase the driving force for Cl^- secretion. In the original recording, CFTR-mediated Cl^- secretion is evidenced by an increase in lumen-negative V_{te} and I_{sc} that is further augmented by cholinergic Ca^{2+}-dependent co-activation with carbachol (CCH). **B:** In patients with 'severe' CF genotypes associated with lack of functional CFTR, cAMP- and Ca^{2+}-dependent Cl^- secretory responses are absent and activation commonly results in inverse lumen-positive responses reflecting luminal K^+ secretion. **C:** In patients with at least one 'mild' CFTR mutation with residual Cl^- channel function, the original tracing shows an attenuated Cl^- secretory response to cAMP stimulation (i.e. lumen negative) and a biphasic response to cholinergic co-activation. Detection of residual CFTR function by ICM is associated with a 'milder' disease phenotype including pancreatic sufficiency (PS). Adopted from Hirtz et al., 2004.

- activation of adenylate cyclase elevating intracellular cAMP, and
- activation of basolateral K^+ channels increasing the driving force for luminal Cl^- secretion

(Roth et al., 2011). This study demonstrated that ICM is sensitive to detect pharmacological activation of residual function of mutant CFTR in native rectal tissues from patients with a large spectrum of CF genotypes.

Small molecule CFTR modulators, developed over the past two decades to restore CFTR function and thus treat the underlying CF defect, showed beneficial effects on lung function and other clinical outcomes in clinical trials, which led to the approval of several CFTR modulator combination therapies for a growing number of patients with CF. However, these trials also showed that patients with the same *CFTR* genotypes treated with CFTR modulators showed heterogeneous responses in clinical outcomes, suggesting that sensitive biomarkers of CFTR function may be important to study the degree of functional rescue of *CFTR* mutations by different CFTR modulators (Graeber et al., 2021). A real world study with the first approved CFTR modulator ivacaftor demonstrated that ICM is sensitive to detect *in vivo* activation of CFTR in individual CF patients with a G551D mutation

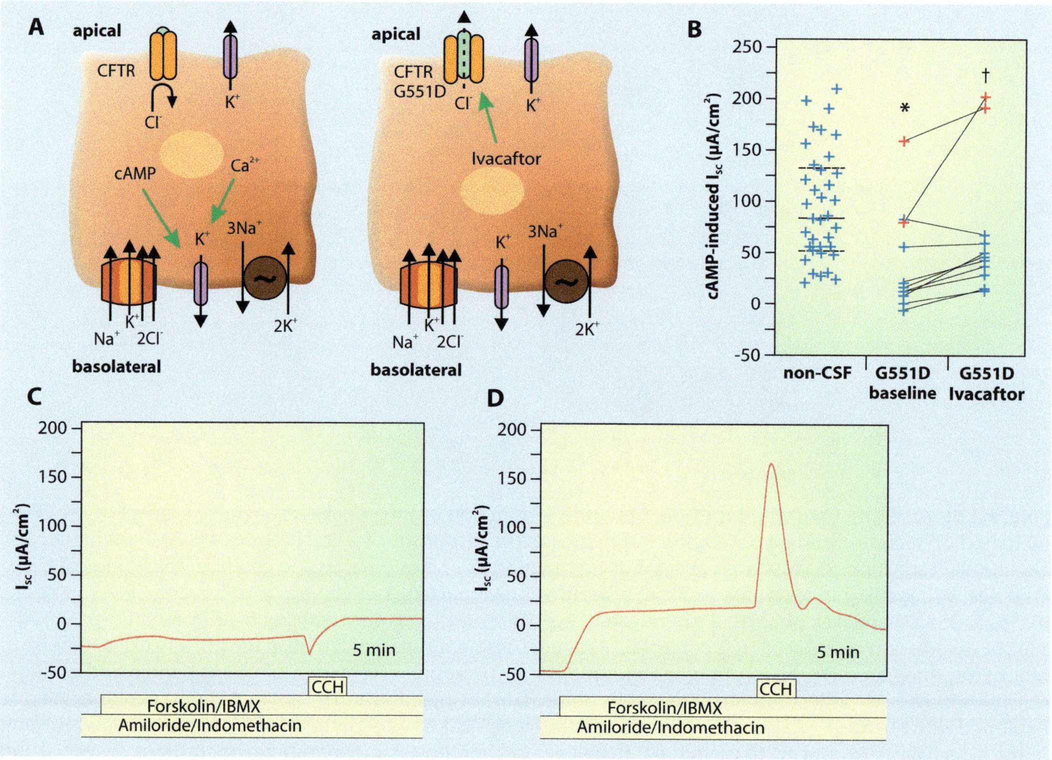

Figure 2.7: Intestinal current measurements (ICM) are sensitive to detect activation of mutant CFTR function in p.Gly551Asp CF patients after initiation of ivacaftor therapy. **A**: Ivacaftor potentiates CFTR-mediated Cl^- secretion by direct activation of the CFTR Cl^- channel. **B**: Summary of cAMP-induced short circuit current (I_{sc}) in rectal biopsies from non-CF individuals (n=37) and p.Gly551Asp patients with CF (n=12) with exocrine pancreatic insufficiency (black dots) or pancreatic sufficiency (red dots) at baseline and after initiation of ivacaftor therapy. **C+D**: Original recordings of sequential effects of cAMP-induced (100 µmol/L 3-isobutyl-1-methylxanthine [IBMX] and 1 µmol/L forskolin, basolateral) and carbachol (CCH)-induced (100 µmol/L, basolateral) I_{sc} in rectal biopsy tissues from a p.Gly551Asp patient with CF (p.Gly551Asp/p.Phe508del) at baseline (**C**) and the same patient with CF after starting ivacaftor therapy (**D**). Experiments were performed in the presence of amiloride and indomethacin. Solid lines represent the group median; dashed lines represent 25th and 75th percentile. *p<0.001 compared with non-CF controls, and †p<0.001 compared with p.Gly551asp CF patients at baseline. Modified after Graeber et al., Am J Respir Crit Care Med. 2015.

(☞ Figure 2.7A; Graeber et al., 2015). In this study, ICM detected activation of CFTR-mediated chloride secretion to a mean level of ~50% of normal CFTR function (☞ Figure 2.7B). Further, lumacaftor-ivacaftor as the first CFTR modulator combination therapy approved for p.Phe508del homozygous CF patients showed a partial rescue of CFTR activity in ICM to levels of ~20% of normal CFTR function (Graeber et al., 2018; Masson et al., 2019). Interestingly, ICM detected improvements in CFTR function even in patients without short-term improvement in FEV1% predicted after initiation of lumacaftor-ivacaftor treatment (Graeber et al., 2018). These findings support the potential of sensitive biomarkers of CFTR function to measure the effect of CFTR modulator therapies on the CF basic defect to enhance personalized medicine in CF. In this context, ICM could be used for quantitative comparison of efficacy of functional correction to select the most effective CFTR modulator combination for patients with common *CFTR* mutations, as well as to identify potentially effective CFTR modulators for patients with rare *CFTR* genotypes (Graeber et al., 2021).

In summary, the ICM technique originally developed by physiologists to elucidate the ion transport pathophysiology in the CF intestine is now available and ready for use in the clinical arena as a sensitive biomarker of CFTR function that can be applied for diagnostic workup of patients with equivocal diagnosis, characterization of *CFTR* mutations with unknown functional consequences and as a sensitive endpoint in preclinical and clinical testing of mutation-specific therapies for CF.

2.4. Primary cystic fibrosis intestinal organoids

Jeffrey M. Beekman

2.4.1. What are organoids?

The last decade showed a strong increase in the use of patient-derived three-dimensional (3D) organoid models for preclinical studies focusing on biology, drug development or individualized medicine applications. Organoids derived from adult stem cells (ASC) proved highly valuable to study key aspects of disease and treatments that aim to restore CFTR function such as CFTR modulators.

Organoids are self-renewing and self-organizing multicellular structures of different cell subsets that capture spatial and functional features of tissues *in vivo* (Lancaster and Knoblich, 2014; Clevers, 2016). These structures require three-dimensional extracellular matrices and defined factors that control self-renewal and differentiation. Organoids can be grown from pluripotent stem cells such as embryonic and induced pluripotent stem cells (iPSC), which enable the generation of organoids containing cells from all germ layers. Alternatively, lineage-committed adult stem cells (ASC) that are derived from tissues post-birth are used to grow organoids that in most cases consist of epithelial cell populations that are found in the original tissues. By recapitulating human tissue more appropriately than transformed cell lines, these models offer new opportunities for disease modeling and therapeutic development.

The first ASC-derived human organoid culture was based on protocols by Sato et al. (2009; 2011), which were initially discovered for mouse intestinal epithelium and then adapted to human intestine and epithelial cells from other organs. Currently, many protocols have been established which enable long-term growth and directed differentiation of tissue-resident epithelial subsets, and biobanked organoid collections are available (e.g at https://huborganoids.nl) for research (Kim et al., 2020).

One exciting new opportunity that ASC-derived organoids that can be grown from easy-to-access tissues is the establishment of large data collections in which individual *in vitro* data can directly be matched with *in vivo* clinical data. Such comparisons are important to validate *in vitro* models as living biomarkers to assist clinical decision making in the context of patient care. Additionally, such clinically-validated *in vitro* models also facilitate a better interpretation and prioritization of biological pathways and interventions thereof and likely improve the translation of findings from the preclinical to the clinical domain.

2.4.2. Organoid swelling as measure of transepithelial ion transport

The original organoid culture protocol produces epithelial organoids that have the apical membrane oriented towards a single lumen. Under standard culture conditions used to expand organoids, healthy control organoid lumens are filled with fluids and have a cystic, spherical appearance (Sato et al., 2011; ☞ Figure 2.8). The fluids in the organoid lumen are actively regulated and can be stimulated through addition of known agonists of epithelial ion and fluid transport (Dekkers et al., 2013; ☞ Figure 2.9). This causes the organoid lumen to increase in size, which leads to subsequent swelling of the whole organoid structure as function of time. Dekkers et al. (2013) showed that CF intestinal organoids have clear phenotypic differences when compared to non-CF counterparts (Dekkers et al., 2013; 2016; ☞ Figure 2.9). The CF organoid lumen volume under standard culture conditions is strongly reduced, leading to visually more condense and irregular organoid structures (☞ Figure 2.10). Additionally, CF organoids show strongly reduced or absent swelling responses upon forskolin stimulation, consistent with reduced or absence of luminal ion and fluid transport (☞ Figure 2.9). Up until now, the forskolin-induced swelling (FIS) of human, mouse and ferret intestinal organoids appears completely CFTR dependent (Dekkers et al., 2013; Schwank et al., 2013; Sun et al., 2019). FIS is inhibited by CFTR inhibitors in healthy control organoids, is absent in organoids containing *CFTR* mutations that lead to non-functional CFTR (class I mutations) and can be reintroduced by CFTR modulators (☞ Figure 2.9) or gene-editing in a *CFTR*-genotype dependent manner.

Direct measures of ion transport in Ussing chambers and organoid swelling correlate (Zomer-van Ommen et al., 2018; Liu et al., 2020). One advantage of phenotypic swelling assays over more classic approaches that measure ion transport directly (e.g. in Ussing chambers, ☞ Chapter 2.3.) is the relative simplicity of the well-plate assay format and reliability on standard microscopy equipment that is available at most research institutes. A clear difference between both models is that fluid secretion in organoids is eventually limited by the physical boundaries of the organoid structure, which may affect fluid secretion differently between both systems. Despite such differences, agonist-induced size increase of organoids as functional assay has now been widely adapted as a measure for epithe-

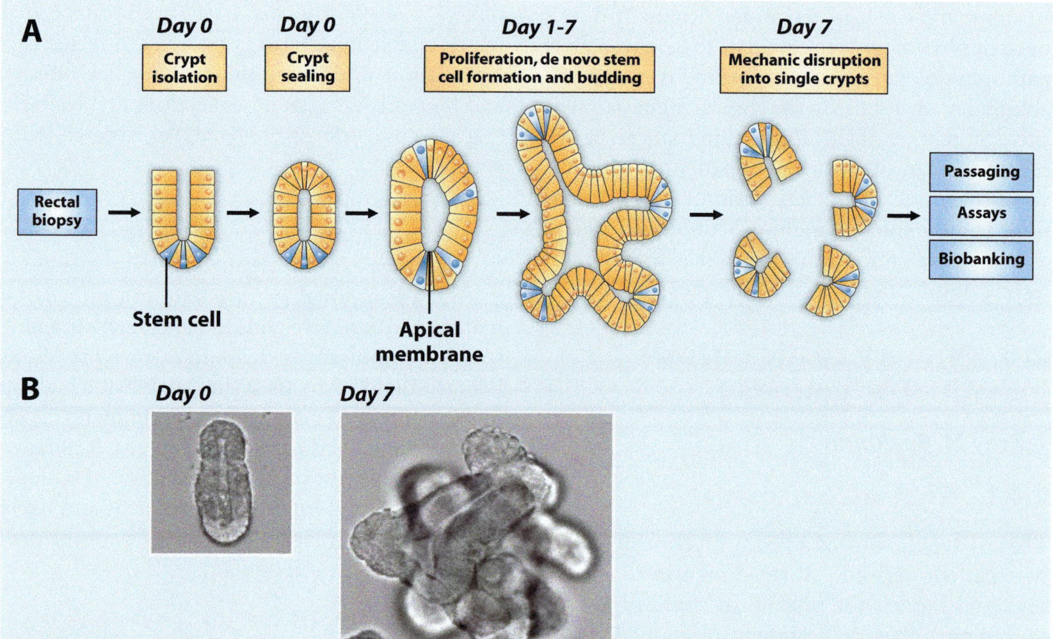

Figure 2.8: Schematic overview of organoid culturing. **A**: Isolated crypts from rectal biopsies self-organize into 3D epithelial structures that recapitulate essential features of the in vivo tissue architecture. **B**: Example microscopy image of an organoid 1 day or 7 days after passaging. Scale bar 30 µm. Modified from a figure in Dekkers et al., 2013b.

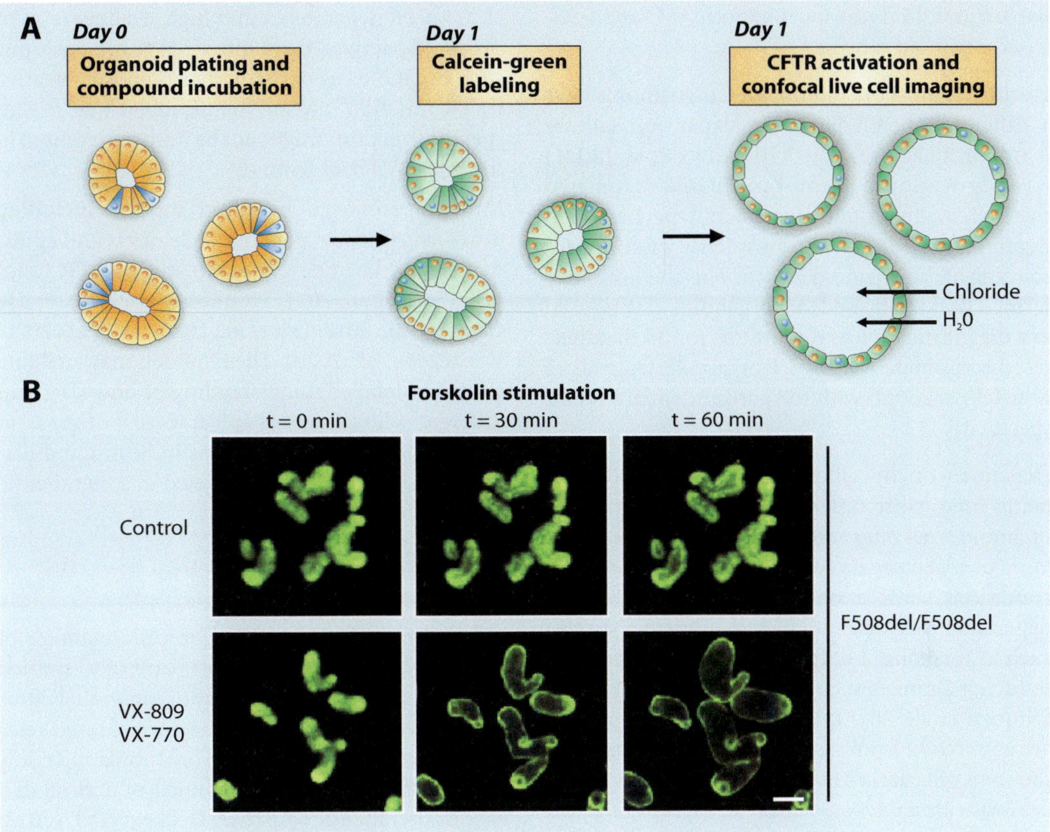

Figure 2.9: Functional CFTR measurements in organoids. **A**: Schematic representation of the 2-day assay to measure forskolin-induced organoid swelling. **B**: Confocal images of calcein-green labeled F508del homozygous organoids with or without treatment of ivacaftor (VX-770) and lumacaftor (VX-809) at the indicated time points of forskolin stimulation. Scale bar 100 μm. Modified from a figure in Dekkers et al., 2013b.

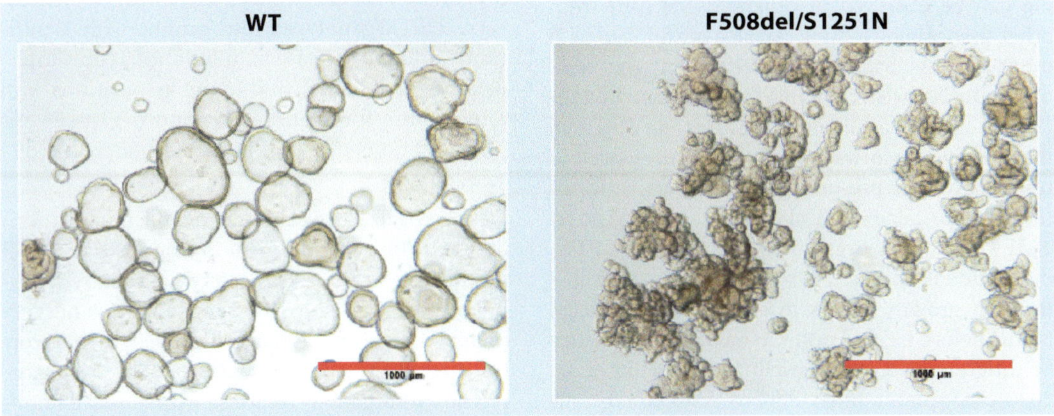

Figure 2.10: Colorectal organoid cultures of a healthy control (left) or person with CF having p.Phe508del/ p.Ser1251Asn CFTR mutations (right) have altered fluid secretion phenotypes in their lumen.

lial ion and fluid transport in both ASC and PSC-based organoid models.

Healthy control organoids and CF organoids have a different phenotype under expansion culture conditions (Figures 2.9+2.10). Cuyx et al. (2021) recently developed a semi-quantitative automated method to quantitate this phenotype based on organoid roundness and low intensity fluorescent staining of the organoid lumen. This methodology termed ROMA showed that organoids may be used as a diagnostic tool, as the authors found that their test discriminated all 167 CF organoids from all 22 non-CF organoids with 100 percent sensitivity and specificity.

Dependent on the cell source and culture protocols being used, clear differences can be observed in organoid swell rates and responses to agonists. Colonic or rectal organoids under expansion culture conditions show a very rapid and fully CFTR-dependent response to cAMP-inducing stimuli such as forskolin, but hardly respond to calcium-inducing agonists such as carbachol (Zomer-van Ommen et al., 2018). When intestinal organoids are withdrawn from stem cell growth factors, both the stem cell marker LGR-5 and CFTR expression are lost within days as well as the basolateral chloride co-transporter (NKCC-1). This is paralleled by reduced forskolin-induced swelling and appearance of mucus-rich goblet cells.

In contrast, non-CFTR dependent organoid swelling can be observed in organoids derived from other tissues and swelling can also be induced with other agonists. Sachs et al. (2019) compared agonist-induced swelling of individually-matched intestinal and airway organoid cultures and observed that specifically airway organoid cultures swell in response to Eact, presumably through activation of the calcium-dependent chloride channel Ano-1/TMEM16a. Nasal organoids can swell in a CFTR-independent manner, which can be controlled through growth factors in the culture medium. Nevertheless, CF and non-CF nasal organoids can be differentiated in the swelling assay (Liu et al., 2020). In general, other PSC or ASC-based non-intestinal organoids including urine-derived kidney organoids (or tubuloids) show reduced swell rates compared to intestinal organoids under organoid expansion conditions (McCauley et al., 2017; Schutgens et al., 2019; Liu et al., 2020). This clear CFTR dependency and high swelling rates of organoids derived from intestinal tissue positions such organoids as particularly suited for sensitive CFTR function measurements, albeit that tissue-specific functions might not be fully represented in the intestinal background.

Multiple epithelial organoid models including those from airway, pancreas, bile ducts and epididymis have been developed to study CFTR function (Sato et al., 2011; Hohwieler et al., 2017; Mc Cauley et al., 2017; Leir et al., 2020; Liu et al., 2020; Verstegen et al., 2020). These models may facilitate a further detailed understanding of how CFTR in different cellular subsets and epithelial origins can coordinate epithelial functions in health and disease, and how this can be targeted in a therapeutic context.

2.4.3. Exploring organoids as living biomarker

Currently, the FIS assay of colorectal organoids of people with CF is the most carefully studied organoid model in the context of individual clinical disease. A series of studies have explored relations between FIS of intestinal organoids and clinical phenotype, both in the context of natural disease or therapeutic response. Dekkers et al. (2013; 2016) showed correlations between organoid FIS and other biomarkers of CFTR function (intestinal current measurements and sweat chloride concentration). Follow-up studies demonstrated that organoid FIS could stratify people with CF with diverse *CFTR* genotypes into groups with significantly different disease manifestations (deWinter-deGroot et al., 2018) and found associations with rate of lung function decline and organ-specific manifestations of CF in liver and pancreatic disease.

Dekkers et al. (2016) also showed the first relations between clinical and organoid responses to CFTR modulators at the *CFTR* genotype level by studying average clinical trial responses and genotype-matched organoids isolated from people that were not directly involved in the clinical study. This correlation of organoid response with clinically non-significant and significant treatment groups led to a first indication of the amount of organoid response that would be needed to show *in vivo* efficacy. Recently, such relations have been independently validated by Ramalho et al. (2021) who found a slightly higher correlation between *CFTR* genotype-specific responses *in vitro* and *in vivo* as compared to Dekkers. Similar observation are also being made with organoids by others derived from the upper airways (Liu et al., 2020), showing also potential for organoid models based on upper respiratory epithelium for selection of drug responders.

In both above mentioned studies of Dekkers and Ramalho, intestinal organoids were also used to select CFTR modulators for people with rare *CFTR* genotypes for whom benefit of CFTR modulators had not yet been demonstrated in clinical studies. Berkers et al. (2019; 2020) studied a larger set of correlations between organoids and individually matched CFTR modulator response *in vivo*. This report focused on people having various *CFTR* genotypes (yet mostly *CFTR* gating mutations) who received different CFTR modulator treatments (e.g. ivacaftor or curcumin/genistein) with clear differences in average efficacy in the study population. Organoid responses were found to correlate both to changes in pulmonary function (percent predicted forced expiry volume at 1 sec) and sweat chloride concentrations. Importantly, the clinical endpoints did not correlate in this study, presumably due to larger contribution of non-CFTR dependent factors on the outcomes of these endpoints as compared to the organoid outcomes. This inability to consistently link different clinical endpoints within individuals complicates the accurate recognition of true clinical responders and therefore thresholds for the organoid test were not defined in this study. Later studies in more homogeneous patient populations (p.Phe508del/p.Ala 445Glu or p.Phe508del/p.Phe508del) and treatment conditions (lumacaftor/ivacaftor) did also not show individual correlations with organoid-based measurements (or any other endpoints or biomarkers of CFTR function; Berkers et al., 2020; Graeber et al., 2020).

These data demonstrate that the interpretation of individual data in short term and small scale clinical studies remains difficult. Even when intestinal or other tissue-derived organoids precisely estimate *in vivo* tissue specific CFTR functions, this only partially captures the complexity of individual disease that is influenced by many additional non-CFTR dependent factors.

Collectively, the current studies show that intestinal organoids and potentially other organoid models can help to discriminate between CF and non-CF, disease expression within CF and therapeutic response to CFTR modulators. Future studies should further explore relevant thresholds of organoid observations in the context of (long-term) natural disease and treatment response, how this is different between various tissue-derived organoid models and how such models should be optimally used with other individual characteristics to enable more accurate predictions of long-term individual disease progression or therapeutic benefit.

2.5. Immunochemical CFTR protein analysis in patients' tissues

Anna-Maria Dittrich, Peter Braubach, Danny Jonigk, Frauke Stanke

CFTR can be visualized in human tissues by immunocytochemistry or western-blot using highly specific antibodies directed against CFTR (Kälin et al., 1999). In contrast to earlier reports (Mall et al., 2004), careful *ex vivo* analysis of patient's tissue has now repeatedly shown that F508del-CFTR can reach the apical membrane (Kreda et al., 2005) and can be fully glycosylated (van Barneveld et al., 2010) in respiratory (Kreda et al., 2005) or gastrointestinal (van Barneveld et al., 2010) tissue. This partially correct CFTR trafficking for mutants such as Phe508del CFTR is consistent with the observation that residual CFTR activity can be detected among p.Phe508del *CFTR* homozygotes (Bronsveld et al., 2001; Sermet-Gaudelus et al., 2002). Apart from Phe508del CFTR, few CFTR mutants have been directly visualized from patients' tissues (van Barneveld et al., 2008; Schucht et al., 2019).

Immunocytochemistry and western blot are complementary techniques that both can answer different questions in the context of whether and how CFTR modulators work: immunocytochemistry allows the characterisation of cell types that do express CFTR whereby ciliated cells, the rare ionocytes (Plasschaert et al., 2018) and the more frequent secretory cells that dominate airway CFTR expression and function (Okuda et al., 2021) can be differentiated (☞ Figure 2.11).

In contrast, western-blot analysis permits the visualization of CFTR glyco-isoforms which is a surro-

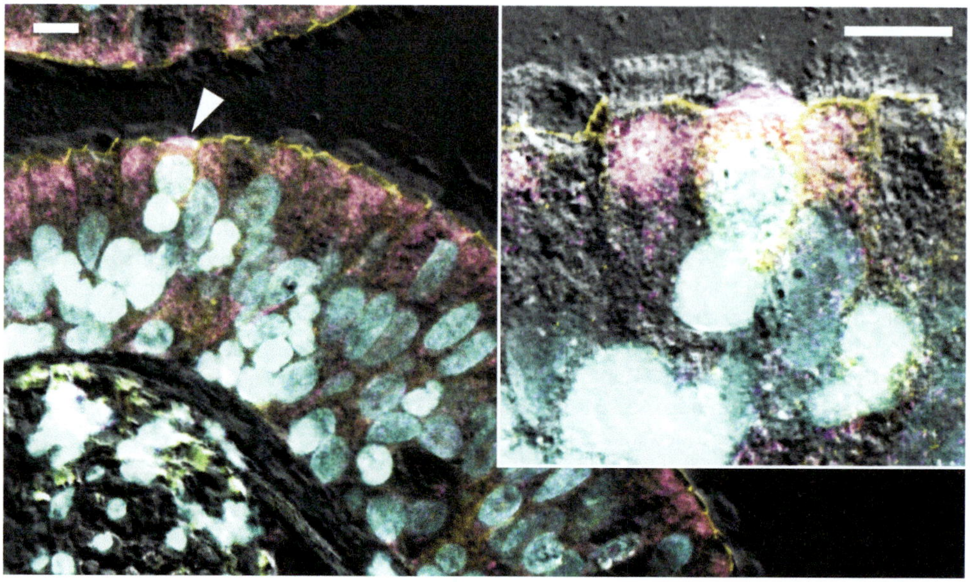

Figure 2.11: Ionocytes (arrowhead) are rare, specialized cells of the bronchial epithelium with an extremely high expression of CFTR. This image shows a typical ionocyte with apical CFTR expression (magenta) between ciliated epithelial cells. Bronchial epithelial tight junctions are marked with ZO1 (yellow), nuclei with DAPI (cyan) on DIC background (gray). Scalebars are 10 µm each. Antibodies used in this experiment were CFTR 596 (Chapel Hill Antibody distribution program 1:400, detected with Alexa 555 1:200) and ZO1 (Abcam ab190085 1:2,000, detected with Alexa 488) with DAPI (Zytovision) as nuclear counterstain.

gate parameter for the efficiency of CFTR trafficking to the apical membrane: CFTR glycosylation is initiated in the ER while core extension, elongation and capping of glycosylation chains occur throughout the Golgi and trans-Golgi network. The polypeptide chain is formed in the endoplasmatic reticulum (CFTR band A) and its mannose-rich core-glycosylated form (CFTR band B) needs to be conveyed to and bypass through the Golgi complex to undergo further trimming and elongation steps before it can reach the apical membrane as complex glycosylated protein (CFTR band C; ☞ Figure 2.12). In other words, the proportion of band B and band C CFTR for wild-type and mutant CFTR can help to understand whether a therapeutic intervention increases CFTR maturation in patients' tissue. We have noticed that the signature of glyco-isoforms differs from patient to patient and that upon triple therapy with elexacaftor/tezacaftor/ivacaftor, any of the following changes in CFTR glyco-isoform ratios can be observed (☞ Figure 2.12): no change in CFTR glyco-isoform (patient P1), a decrease of band C CFTR (P2) or an increase of CFTR band C (P3).

Apart from the canonical processing of complex glycosylated membrane proteins in polarized epithelial cells, CFTR band B can bypass the Golgi complex directly and use the Golgi reassembly-stacking protein (GRASP)-mediated pathway that has been identified as an alternative route for Phe508del CFTR maturation under conditions of ER stress in mostly non-polar cells that express CFTR heterologously (Yoo et al., 2002; Gee et al., 2011). It remains to be clarified whether these or other alternative routes of protein glycosylation, defined by one or more out of 14 pathways that together rely on a total of 173 glycosyltransferases (Schjoldager et al., 2020), can assist in the generation and/or trafficking of CFTR glyco-isoforms to the apical membrane in patient's tissues *in vivo* and whether or not these maturation pathways can be modified by small-molecule therapeutics directed at CFTR.

2.6. References

Accurso FJ, Van Goor F, Zha J, Stone AJ, Dong Q, Ordonez CL, Rowe SM, Clancy JP, Konstan MW, Hoch HE, Heltshe SL, Ramsey BW, Campbell PW, Ashlock MA. Sweat chloride as a biomarker of CFTR activity:

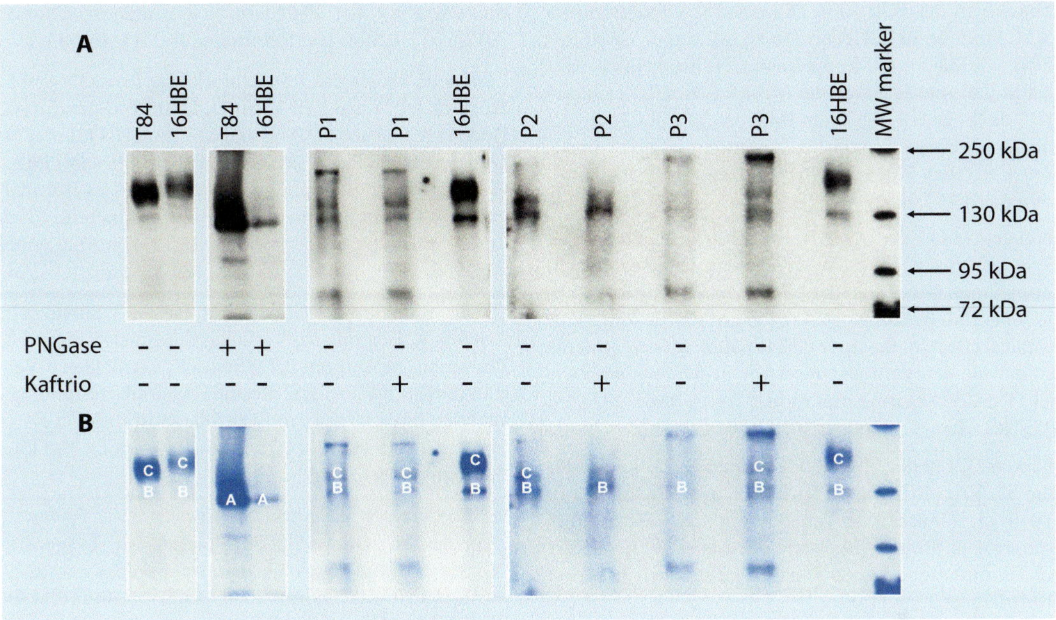

Figure 2.12: Detection of CFTR glycoisoforms by western-blot from rectal suction biopsies derived from CF patients prior to and after treatment with elexacaftor/tezacaftor/ivacaftor. **A**: Biomaterial from epithelial model cell lines T84 (intestinal, cancer), 16HBE14o- (tracheal, virus-immortalised, 16HBE) and three CF patients who participated in the post-approval trial with elexacaftor/tezacaftor/ivacaftor (Kaftriofacts) are shown. SDS-rich whole cell lysates were prepared using Laemmli buffer (2% SDS, 10% glycerol) to homogenize cell layers of ALI cultures. To detect CFTR, lysates were incubated for 30 min at 37 °C prior to loading on a denaturing 6% polyacrylamide gel at 4 °C for 18 h until the 72 kDa size marker band approached end of the acrylamide matrix. Transfer to a nitrocellulose (Hybond C, GE Healthcare, Chicago, IL, USA) membrane was done immersed in an ice bath at 0 °C for 18 h. Starting Block Buffer (Thermo Fisher Scientific, Waltham, MA, USA) was used for blocking for 2 h at room temperature. CFTR detection was done using four CFTR monoclonal antibodies provided by T. Jensen, Chapel Hill via the antibody distribution program hosted by the CF foundation (Abs 217, 660, 570, 596) in a mixture of 1:1:1:1. Depending on signal intensity, two different HRP substrate solutions (SuperSignal West Pico or SuperSignal West Femto, Thermo Fisher Scientific) were applied onto membranes. In model cell lines T84 and 16HBE14o-, CFTR band A was obtained using PNGase. **B**: CFTR glyco-isoforms. The polypeptide chain is formed in the endoplasmatic reticulum (CFTR band A); subsequently, glycosyl residues are added to form core-glycosylated proteins prior to ER exit (CFTR band B) and finally mature complex glycosylated glycoproteins processed in the Golgi reach the apical membrane (CFTR band C).

proof of concept and ivacaftor clinical trial data. J Cyst Fibros. 2014;13:139-47. doi: 10.1016/j.jcf.2013.09.007.

Accurso FJ, Rowe SM, Clancy JP, Boyle MP, Dunitz JM, Durie PR, Sagel SD, Hornick DB, Konstan MW, Donaldson SH, Moss RB, Pilewski JM, Rubenstein RC, Uluer AZ, Aitken ML, Freedman SD, Rose LM, Mayer-Hamblett N, Dong Q, Zha J, Stone AJ, Olson ER, Ordoñez CL, Campbell PW, Ashlock MA, Ramsey BW. Effect of VX-770 in persons with cystic fibrosis and the G551D-CFTR mutation. N Engl J Med. 2010;363:1991-2003. doi: 10.1056/NEJMoa0909825.

Bagheri-Hanson A, Nedwed S, Rueckes-Nilges C, Naehrlich L. Intestinal current measurement versus nasal potential difference measurements for diagnosis of cystic fibrosis: a case-control study. BMC Pulm Med. 2014;14:156. doi: 10.1186/1471-2466-14-156.

Behm JK, Hagiwara G, Lewiston NJ, Quinton PM, Wine JJ. Hyposecretion of β-adrenergically induced sweating in CF heterozygotes. Pediatr Res 1987;22:271-276. doi: 10.1203/00006450-198709000-00007.

Bergamini G, Tridello G, Calcaterra E, Ceri S, Tagliasacchi M, Bianchi F, Monti F, Masciadri A, Laudanna E, Peserico D, Sorio E, Esposito V, Leal T, Assael BM, Sorio C, Melotti P. Ratiometric sweat secretion optical test in cystic fibrosis, carriers and healthy subjects. J Cyst Fibros 2018;17:186-9. doi: 10.1016/j.jcf.2017.12.003.

Berkers G, van Mourik P, Vonk AM, Kruisselbrink E, Dekkers JF, de Winter-de Groot KM, Arets HGM,

Marck-van der Wilt REP, Dijkema JS, Vanderschuren MM, Houwen RHJ, Heijerman HGM, van de Graaf EA, Elias SG, Majoor CJ, Koppelman GH, Roukema J, Bakker M, Janssens HM, van der Meer R, Vries RGJ, Clevers HC, de Jonge HR, Beekman JM, van der Ent CK. Rectal organoids enable personalized treatment of cystic fibrosis. Cell Rep. 2019;26:1701-1708.e3. doi: 10.1016/j.celrep.2019.01.068.

Berkers G, van der Meer R, van Mourik P, Vonk AM, Kruisselbrink E, Suen SW, Heijerman HG, Majoor CJ, Koppelman GH, Roukema J, Janssens HM, de Rijke YB, Kemper EM, Beekman JM, van der Ent CK, de Jonge HR. Clinical effects of the three CFTR potentiator treatments curcumin, genistein and ivacaftor in patients with the CFTR-S1251N gating mutation. J Cyst Fibros. 2020;19: 955-961. doi: 10.1016/j.jcf.2020.04.014.

Berkers G, van der Meer R, Heijerman H, Beekman JM, Boj SF, Vries RGJ, van Mourik P, Doyle JR, Audhya P, Yuan ZJ, Kinnman N, van der Ent CK. Lumacaftor/ivacaftor in people with cystic fibrosis with an A455E-CFTR mutation. J Cyst Fibros. 2021;20:761-767. doi: 10.1016/j.jcf.2020.11.007.

Bronsveld I, Mekus F, Bijman J, Ballmann M, Greipel J, Hundrieser J, Halley DJ, Laabs U, Busche R, De Jonge HR, Tümmler B, Veeze HJ. Residual chloride secretion in intestinal tissue of deltaF508 homozygous twins and siblings with cystic fibrosis. The European CF Twin and Sibling Study Consortium. Gastroenterology. 2000;119: 32-40. doi: 10.1053/gast.2000.8524.

Bronsveld I, Mekus F, Bijman J, Ballmann M, de Jonge HR, Laabs U, Halley DJ, Ellemunter H, Mastella G, Thomas S, Veeze HJ, Tümmler B. Chloride conductance and genetic background modulate the cystic fibrosis phenotype of Delta F508 homozygous twins and siblings. J Clin Invest. 2001;108:1705-15. doi: 10.1172/JCI12108.

CFFT Therapeutics Development Network Coordinating Center, Rowe S, Clancy JP, Beamer J. Standardization of measurement of nasal membrane transepithelial potential difference (NPD) – EDC and perfusion or perfusion-free probe. Protocol 528.00, 2009.

Char JE, Dunn C, Davies Z, Milla C, Moss RB, Wine JJ. The magnitude of ivacaftor effects on fluid secretion via R117H-CFTR channels: Human in vivo measurements. PLoS One. 2017;12:e0175486. doi: 10.1371/journal.pone.0175486.

Clancy JP, Rowe SM, Accurso FJ, Aitken ML, Amin RS, Ashlock MA, Ballmann M, Boyle MP, Bronsveld I, Campbell PW, De Boeck K, Donaldson SH, Dorkin HL, Dunitz JM, Durie PR, Jain M, Leonard A, McCoy KS, Moss RB, Pilewski JM, Rosenbluth DB, Rubenstein RC, Schechter MS, Botfield M, Ordoñez CL, Spencer-Green GT, Vernillet L, Wisseh S, Yen K, Konstan MW. Results of a phase IIa study of VX-809, an investigational CFTR corrector compound, in subjects with cystic fibrosis homozygous for the F508del-CFTR mutation. Thorax. 2012;67:12-8. doi: 10.1136/thoraxjnl-2011-200393.

Clancy JP, Szczesniak RD, Ashlock MA, Ernst SE, Fan L, Hornick DB, Karp PH, Khan U, Lymp J, Ostmann AJ, Rezayat A, Starner TD, Sugandha SP, Sun H, Quinney N, Donaldson SH, Rowe SM, Gabriel SE. Multicenter intestinal current measurements in rectal biopsies from CF and non-CF subjects to monitor CFTR function. PLoS One. 2013;8:e73905. doi: 10.1371/journal.pone.0073905.

Cuyx S, Ramalho AS, Corthout N, Fieuws S, Fürstová E, Arnauts K, Ferrante M, Verfaillie C, Munck S, Boon M, Proesmans M, Dupont L, De Boeck K, Vermeulen F; Belgian Organoid Project. Rectal organoid morphology analysis (ROMA) as a promising diagnostic tool in cystic fibrosis. Thorax. 2021;76:1146-1149. doi: 10.1136/thoraxjnl-2020-216368.

De Boeck K, Wilschanski M, Castellani C, Taylor C, Cuppens H, Dodge J, Sinaasappel M; Diagnostic Working Group. Cystic fibrosis: terminology and diagnostic algorithms. Thorax. 2006;61:627-35. doi: 10.1136/thx.2005.043539.

De Boeck K, Kent L, Davies J, Derichs N, Amaral M, Rowe SM, Middleton P, de Jonge H, Bronsveld I, Wilschanski M, Melotti P, Danner-Boucher I, Boerner S, Fajac I, Southern K, de Nooijer RA, Bot A, de Rijke Y, de Wachter E, Leal T, Vermeulen F, Hug MJ, Rault G, Nguyen-Khoa T, Barreto C, Proesmans M, Sermet-Gaudelus I; European Cystic Fibrosis Society Clinical Trial Network Standardisation Committee. CFTR biomarkers: time for promotion to surrogate end-point. Eur Respir J. 2013;41:203-16. doi: 10.1183/09031936.00057512.

De Jonge HR, Ballmann M, Veeze H, Bronsveld I, Stanke F, Tümmler B, Sinaasappel M. Ex vivo CF diagnosis by intestinal current measurements (ICM) in small aperture, circulating Ussing chambers. J Cyst Fibros 2004;3 Suppl 2:159-163. doi: 10.1016/j.jcf.2004.05.034.

de Winter-de Groot KM, Janssens HM, van Uum RT, Dekkers JF, Berkers G, Vonk A, Kruisselbrink E, Oppelaar H, Vries R, Clevers H, Houwen RHJ, Escher JC, Elias SG, de Jonge HR, de Rijke YB, Tiddens HAWM, van der Ent CK, Beekman JM. Stratifying infants with cystic fibrosis for disease severity using intestinal organoid swelling as a biomarker of CFTR function. Eur Respir J. 2018;52:1702529. doi: 10.1183/13993003.02529-2017.

Dekkers JF, Wiegerinck CL, de Jonge HR, Bronsveld I, Janssens HM, de Winter-de Groot KM, Brandsma AM, de Jong NW, Bijvelds MJ, Scholte BJ, Nieuwenhuis EE, van den Brink S, Clevers H, van der Ent CK, Middendorp S, Beekman JM. A functional CFTR assay using primary cystic fibrosis intestinal organoids. Nat Med. 2013;19: 939-45. doi: 10.1038/nm.3201.

Dekkers JF, Berkers G, Kruisselbrink E, Vonk A, de Jonge HR, Janssens HM, Bronsveld I, van de Graaf EA, Nieuwenhuis EE, Houwen RH, Vleggaar FP, Escher JC, de Rijke YB, Majoor CJ, Heijerman HG, de Winter-de Groot KM, Clevers H, van der Ent CK, Beekman JM. Characterizing responses to CFTR-modulating drugs using rectal organoids derived from subjects with cystic fibrosis. Sci Transl Med. 2016;8:344ra84. doi: 10.1126/scitranslmed.aad8278.

Derichs N, Sanz J, Von Kanel T, Stolpe C, Zapf A, Tümmler B, Gallati S, Ballmann M. Intestinal current measurement for diagnostic classification of patients with questionable cystic fibrosis: validation and reference data. Thorax. 2010;65:594-9. doi: 10.1136/thx.2009.125088.

Durno C, Corey M, Zielenski J, Tullis E, Tsui LC, Durie P. Genotype and phenotype correlations in patients with cystic fibrosis and pancreatitis. Gastroenterology. 2002;123:1857-64. doi: 10.1053/gast.2002.37042.

European Cystic Fibrosis Society (ECFS) Diagnostic Network Working Group & Clinical Trials Network, Bronsveld I, Sermet-Gaudelus I. Nasal potential difference (NPD) measurement for diagnosis and clinical trials in cystic fibrosis. NPD_EU001, version 1.7, 2013.

Farrell PM, Rosenstein BJ, White TB, Accurso FJ, Castellani C, Cutting GR, Durie PR, Legrys VA, Massie J, Parad RB, Rock MJ, Campbell PW 3rd; Cystic Fibrosis Foundation. Guidelines for diagnosis of cystic fibrosis in newborns through older adults: Cystic Fibrosis Foundation consensus report. J Pediatr. 2008;153:S4-S14. doi: 10.1016/j.jpeds.2008.05.005.

Gee HY, Noh SH, Tang BL, Kim KH, Lee MG. Rescue of ΔF508-CFTR trafficking via a GRASP-dependent unconventional secretion pathway. Cell. 2011;146:746-60. doi: 10.1016/j.cell.2011.07.021.

Gibson LE, Cooke RE. A test for concentration of electrolytes in sweat in cystic fibrosis of the pancreas utilizing pilocarpine by iontophoresis. Pediatrics 1959;23: 545-549.

Fidler MC, Beusmans J, Panorchan P, Van Goor F. Correlation of sweat chloride and percent predicted FEV(1) in cystic fibrosis patients treated with ivacaftor. J Cyst Fibros 2017;16:41-44. doi: 10.1016/j.jcf.2016.10.002.

Gonska T, Choi P, Stephenson A, Ellis L, Martin S, Solomon M, Dupuis A, Dorfman R, Zielenski J, Ooi CY, Weiser W, Durie PR, Tullis E. Role of cystic fibrosis transmembrane conductance regulator in patients with chronic sinopulmonary disease. Chest. 2012;142:996-1004. doi: 10.1378/chest.11-2543.

Graeber SY, Hug MJ, Sommerburg O, Hirtz S, Hentschel J, Heinzmann A, Dopfer C, Schulz A, Mainz JG, Tümmler B, Mall MA. Intestinal current measurements detect activation of mutant CFTR in patients with cystic fibrosis with the G551D mutation treated with Ivacaftor. Am J Respir Crit Care Med. 2015;192:1252-5. doi: 10.1164/rccm.201507-1271LE.

Graeber SY, Dopfer C, Naehrlich L, Gyulumyan L, Scheuermann H, Hirtz S, Wege S, Mairbäurl H, Dorda M, Hyde R, Bagheri-Hanson A, Rueckes-Nilges C, Fischer S, Mall MA, Tümmler B. Effects of Lumacaftor-Ivacaftor therapy on Cystic Fibrosis Transmembrane Conductance Regulator function in Phe508del homozygous patients with cystic fibrosis. Am J Respir Crit Care Med. 2018;197:1433-1442. doi: 10.1164/rccm.201710-1983OC.

Graeber SY, van Mourik P, Vonk AM, Kruisselbrink E, Hirtz S, van der Ent CK, Mall MA, Beekman JM. Comparison of organoid swelling and *in vivo* biomarkers of CFTR function to determine effects of Lumacaftor-Ivacaftor in patients with cystic fibrosis homozygous for the F508del mutation. Am J Respir Crit Care Med. 2020;202:1589-1592. doi: 10.1164/rccm.202004-1200LE.

Graeber SY, Vitzthum C, Mall MA. Potential of intestinal current measurement for personalized treatment of patients with cystic fibrosis. J Pers Med. 2021;11:384. doi: 10.3390/jpm11050384.

Graeber SY, Vitzthum C, Pallenberg ST, Naehrlich L, Stahl M, Rohrbach A, Drescher M, Minso R, Ringshausen FC, Rueckes-Nilges C, Klajda J, Berges J, Yu Y, Scheuermann H, Hirtz S, Sommerburg O, Dittrich AM, Tümmler B, Mall MA. Effects of Elexacaftor/Tezacaftor/Ivacaftor therapy on CFTR function in patients with cystic fibrosis and one or two *F508del* alleles. Am J Respir Crit Care Med 2021 Dec 22. doi: 10.1164/rccm.202110-2249OC.

Green A, Kirk J, Guidelines Development Group. Guidelines for the performance of the sweat test for the diagnosis of cystic fibrosis. Ann Clin Biochem. 2007;44:25-34. doi: 10.1258/000456307779596011.

Hardcastle J, Hardcastle PT, Taylor CJ, Goldhill J. Failure of cholinergic stimulation to induce a secretory response from the rectal mucosa in cystic fibrosis. Gut 1991;32:1035-1039. doi: 10.1136/gut.32.9.1035.

Hentschel J, Riesener G, Nelle H, Stuhrmann M, Schöner A, Sommerburg O, Fritzsching E, Mall MA, von Eggeling F, Mainz JG. Homozygous *CFTR* mutation M348K in a boy with respiratory symptoms and failure to thrive. Disease-causing mutation or benign alteration? Eur J Pediatr. 2012;171:1039-46. doi: 10.1007/s00431-012-1672-1.

Hirtz S, Gonska T, Seydewitz HH, Thomas J, Greiner P, Kuehr J, Brandis M, Eichler I, Rocha H, Lopes AI, Barreto C, Ramalho A, Amaral MD, Kunzelmann K, Mall M. CFTR Cl- channel function in native human colon correlates with the genotype and phenotype in cystic fibrosis. Gastroenterology. 2004;127:1085-95. doi: 10.1053/j.gastro.2004.07.006.

Hohwieler M, Illing A, Hermann PC, Mayer T, Stockmann M, Perkhofer L, Eiseler T, Antony JS, Müller M, Renz S, Kuo CC, Lin Q, Sendler M, Breunig M, Kleiderman SM, Lechel A, Zenker M, Leichsenring M, Rosendahl J, Zenke M, Sainz B Jr, Mayerle J, Costa IG, Seufferlein T, Kormann M, Wagner M, Liebau S, Kleger A. Human pluripotent stem cell-derived acinar/ductal organoids generate human pancreas upon orthotopic transplantation and allow disease modelling. Gut. 2017; 66:473-486. doi: 10.1136/gutjnl-2016-312423.

Kälin N, Claass A, Sommer M, Puchelle E, Tümmler B. DeltaF508 CFTR protein expression in tissues from patients with cystic fibrosis. J Clin Invest. 1999;103:1379-89. doi: 10.1172/JCI5731.

Kerem E, Hirawat S, Armoni S, Yaakov Y, Shoseyov D, Cohen M, Nissim-Rafinia M, Blau H, Rivlin J, Aviram M, Elfring GL, Northcutt VJ, Miller LL, Kerem B, Wilschanski M. Effectiveness of PTC124 treatment of cystic fibrosis caused by nonsense mutations: a prospective phase II trial. Lancet. 2008;372:719-27. doi: 10.1016/S0140-6736(08)61168-X.

Kim J, Farahmand M, Dunn C, Davies Z, Frisbee E, Milla C, Wine JJ. Evaporimeter and bubble-imaging measures of sweat gland secretion rates. PLoS One. 2016;11: e0165254. doi: 10.1371/journal.pone.0165254.

Kim J, Farahmand M, Dunn C, Milla CE, Horii RI, Thomas EAC, Moss RB, Wine JJ. Sweat rate analysis of ivacaftor potentiation of CFTR in non-CF adults. Sci Rep. 2018;8:16233. doi: 10.1038/s41598-018-34308-8.

Kim J, Koo BK, Knoblich JA. Human organoids: model systems for human biology and medicine. Nat Rev Mol Cell Biol. 2020;21:571-584. doi: 10.1038/s41580-020-0259-3.

Knowles M, Gatzy J, Boucher R. Increased bioelectric potential difference across respiratory epithelia in cystic fibrosis. N Engl J Med 1981;305:1489-95. doi: 10.1056/NEJM198112173052502.

Knowles M, Gatzy J, Boucher R. Relative ion permeability of normal and cystic fibrosis nasal epithelium. J Clin Invest 1983a;71:1410-7. doi: 10.1172/jci110894.

Knowles MR, Stutts MJ, Spock A, Fischer N, Gatzy JT, Boucher RC. Abnormal ion permeation through cystic fibrosis respiratory epithelium. Science. 1983b;221: 1067-70. doi: 10.1126/science.6308769.

Knowles MR, Paradiso AM, Boucher RC. In vivo nasal potential difference: techniques and protocols for assessing efficacy of gene transfer in cystic fibrosis. Hum Gene Ther 1995; 6:445-55. doi: 10.1089/hum.1995.6.4-445.

Kreda SM, Mall M, Mengos A, Rochelle L, Yankaskas J, Riordan JR, Boucher RC. Characterization of wild-type and deltaF508 cystic fibrosis transmembrane regulator in human respiratory epithelia. Mol Biol Cell. 2005;16: 2154-67. doi: 10.1091/mbc.e04-11-1010.

Kunzelmann K, Mall M. Electrolyte transport in the mammalian colon: mechanisms and implications for disease. Physiol Rev. 2002;82:245-89. doi: 10.1152/physrev.00026.2001.

Lancaster MA, Knoblich JA. Organogenesis in a dish: modeling development and disease using organoid technologies. Science. 2014;345:1247125. doi: 10.1126/science.1247125.

Leir SH, Yin S, Kerschner JL, Xia S, Ahmadi S, Bear C, Harris A. An organoid model to assay the role of CFTR in the human epididymis epithelium. Cell Tissue Res. 2020; 381:327-336. doi: 10.1007/s00441-020-03208-7.

Li H, Sheppard DN, Hug MJ. Transepithelial electrical measurements with the Ussing chamber. J Cyst Fibros 2004;3 Suppl 2:123-126. doi: 10.1016/j.jcf.2004.05.026.

Liu Z, Anderson JD, Deng L, Mackay S, Bailey J, Kersh L, Rowe SM, Guimbellot JS. Human nasal epithelial organoids for therapeutic development in cystic fibrosis. Genes (Basel). 2020;11:603. doi: 10.3390/genes 11060603.

Mall M, Bleich M, Schürlein M, Kühr J, Seydewitz HH, Brandis M, Greger R, Kunzelmann K. Cholinergic ion secretion in human colon requires coactivation by cAMP. Am J Physiol. 1998; 275:G1274-81. doi: 10.1152/ajpgi.1998.275.6.G1274.

Mall M, Bleich M, Kuehr J, Brandis M, Greger R, Kunzelmann K. CFTR-mediated inhibition of epithelial Na^+ conductance in human colon is defective in cystic fibrosis. Am J Physiol. 1999; 277:G709-16. doi: 10.1152/ajpgi.1999.277.3.G709.

Mall M, Wissner A, Seydewitz HH, Kuehr J, Brandis M, Greger R, Kunzelmann K. Defective cholinergic $Cl(^-)$ secretion and detection of $K(^+)$ secretion in rectal biopsies from cystic fibrosis patients. Am J Physiol Gastrointest Liver Physiol. 2000;278:G617-24. doi: 10.1152/ajpgi.2000.278.4.G617.

Mall M, Hirtz S, Gonska T, Kunzelmann K. Assessment of CFTR function in rectal biopsies for the diagnosis of cystic fibrosis. J Cyst Fibros 2004;3 Suppl 2:165-169. doi: 10.1016/j.jcf.2004.05.035.

Mall M, Kreda SM, Mengos A, Jensen TJ, Hirtz S, Seydewitz HH, Yankaskas J, Kunzelmann K, Riordan JR, Boucher RC. The DeltaF508 mutation results in loss of CFTR function and mature protein in native human colon. Gastroenterology. 2004;126:32-41. doi: 10.1053/j.gastro.2003.10.049.

Masson A, Schneider-Futschik EK, Baatallah N, Nguyen-Khoa T, Girodon E, Hatton A, Flament T, Le Bourgeois M, Chedevergne F, Bailly C, Kyrilli S, Achimastos

D, Hinzpeter A, Edelman A, Sermet-Gaudelus I. Predictive factors for lumacaftor/ivacaftor clinical response. J Cyst Fibros. 2019;18:368-374. doi: 10.1016/j.jcf.2018.12.011.

McCauley KB, Hawkins F, Serra M, Thomas DC, Jacob A, Kotton DN. Efficient derivation of functional human airway epithelium from pluripotent stem cells via temporal regulation of Wnt signaling. Cell Stem Cell. 2017; 20:844-857. doi: 10.1016/j.stem.2017.03.001.

Middleton PG, Geddes DM, Alton EW. Protocols for in vivo measurement of the ion transport defects in cystic fibrosis nasal epithelium. Eur Respir J. 1994;7:2050-6.

Middleton PG, Mall MA, Drevínek P, Lands LC, Mc Kone EF, Polineni D, Ramsey BW, Taylor-Cousar JL, Tullis E, Vermeulen F, Marigowda G, McKee CM, Moskowitz SM, Nair N, Savage J, Simard C, Tian S, Waltz D, Xuan F, Rowe SM, Jain R; VX17-445-102 Study Group. Elexacaftor-Tezacaftor-Ivacaftor for Cystic Fibrosis with a Single Phe508del Allele. N Engl J Med. 2019;381:1809-1819. doi: 10.1056/NEJMoa1908639.

Minso R, Schulz A, Dopfer C, Alfeis N, Barneveld AV, Makartian-Gyulumyan L, Hansen G, Junge S, Müller C, Ringshausen FCC, Sauer-Heilborn A, Stanke F, Stolpe C, Tamm S, Welte T, Dittrich AM, Tümmler B. Intestinal current measurement and nasal potential difference to make a diagnosis of cases with inconclusive *CFTR* genetics and sweat test. BMJ Open Respir Res. 2020;7:e000736. doi: 10.1136/bmjresp-2020-000736.

Okuda K, Dang H, Kobayashi Y, Carraro G, Nakano S, Chen G, Kato T, Asakura T, Gilmore RC, Morton LC, Lee RE, Mascenik T, Yin WN, Barbosa Cardenas SM, O'Neal YK, Minnick CE, Chua M, Quinney NL, Gentzsch M, Anderson CW, Ghio A, Matsui H, Nagase T, Ostrowski LE, Grubb BR, Olsen JC, Randell SH, Stripp BR, Tata PR, O'Neal WK, Boucher RC. Secretory cells dominate airway CFTR expression and function in human airway superficial epithelia. Am J Respir Crit Care Med. 2021;203:1275-1289. doi: 10.1164/rccm.202008-3198OC.

Ooi CY, Dupuis A, Gonska T, Ellis L, Ni A, Jarvi K, Martin S, Ray P, Steele L, Kortan P, Dorfman R, Solomon M, Zielenski J, Corey M, Tullis E, Durie P. Does integration of various ion channel measurements improve diagnostic performance in cystic fibrosis? Ann Am Thorac Soc. 2014;11:562-70. doi: 10.1513/AnnalsATS.201311-412 OC.

Pallenberg ST, Junge S, Ringshausen FC, Sauer-Heilborn A, Hansen G, Dittrich AM, Tümmler B, Nietert M. CFTR modulation with elexacaftor-tezacaftor-ivacaftor in people with cystic fibrosis assessed by the β-adrenergic sweat rate assay. J Cyst Fibros. 2021;S1569-1993(21) 02107-X. doi: 10.1016/j.jcf.2021.10.005

Plasschaert LW, Zilionis R, Choo-Wing R, Savova V, Knehr J, Roma G, Klein AM, Jaffe AB. A single-cell atlas of the airway epithelium reveals the CFTR-rich pulmonary ionocyte. Nature. 2018;560:377-381. doi: 10.1038/s41586-018-0394-6.

Quinton PM. Chloride impermeability in cystic fibrosis. Nature. 1983;301:421-2. doi: 10.1038/301421a0.

Quinton PM. Cystic fibrosis: lessons from the sweat gland. Physiology (Bethesda). 2007; 22:212-25. doi: 10.1152/physiol.00041.2006.

Quinton P, Molyneux L, Ip W, Dupuis A, Avolio J, Tullis E, Conrad D, Shamsuddin AK, Durie P, Gonska T. β-adrenergic sweat secretion as a diagnostic test for cystic fibrosis. Am J Respir Crit Care Med. 2012;186:732-9. doi: 10.1164/rccm.201205-0922OC.

Ramalho AS, Fürstová E, Vonk AM, Ferrante M, Verfaillie C, Dupont L, Boon M, Proesmans M, Beekman JM, Sarouk I, Vazquez Cordero C, Vermeulen F, De Boeck K; Belgian Organoid Project. Correction of CFTR function in intestinal organoids to guide treatment of cystic fibrosis. Eur Respir J. 2021;57:1902426. doi: 10.1183/13993003.02426-2019.

Ramsey BW, Davies J, McElvaney NG, Tullis E, Bell SC, Drevínek P, Griese M, McKone EF, Wainwright CE, Konstan MW, Moss R, Ratjen F, Sermet-Gaudelus I, Rowe SM, Dong Q, Rodriguez S, Yen K, Ordoñez C, Elborn JS; VX08-770-102 Study Group. A CFTR potentiator in patients with cystic fibrosis and the G551D mutation. N Engl J Med. 2011;365:1663-72. doi: 10.1056/NEJMoa1105185.

Rosenstein BJ, Cutting GR. The diagnosis of cystic fibrosis: a consensus statement. Cystic Fibrosis Foundation Consensus Panel. J Pediatr. 1998;132:589-95. doi: 10.1016/s0022-3476(98)70344-0.

Roth EK, Hirtz S, Duerr J, Wenning D, Eichler I, Seydewitz HH, Amaral MD, Mall MA. The K^+ channel opener 1-EBIO potentiates residual function of mutant CFTR in rectal biopsies from cystic fibrosis patients. PLoS One. 2011;6:e24445. doi: 10.1371/journal.pone.0024445.

Sachs N, Papaspyropoulos A, Zomer-van Ommen DD, Heo I, Böttinger L, Klay D, Weeber F, Huelsz-Prince G, Iakobachvili N, Amatngalim GD, de Ligt J, van Hoeck A, Proost N, Viveen MC, Lyubimova A, Teeven L, Derakhshan S, Korving J, Begthel H, Dekkers JF, Kumawat K, Ramos E, van Oosterhout MF, Offerhaus GJ, Wiener DJ, Olimpio EP, Dijkstra KK, Smit EF, van der Linden M, Jaksani S, van de Ven M, Jonkers J, Rios AC, Voest EE, van Moorsel CH, van der Ent CK, Cuppen E, van Oudenaarden A, Coenjaerts FE, Meyaard L, Bont LJ, Peters PJ, Tans SJ, van Zon JS, Boj SF, Vries RG, Beekman JM, Clevers H. Long-term expanding human airway organoids for disease modeling. EMBO J. 2019;38: e100300. doi: 10.15252/embj.2018100300.

Salinas DB, Peng YH, Horwich B, Wee CP, Frisbee E, Maarek JM. Image-based β-adrenergic sweat rate assay captures minimal cystic fibrosis transmembrane conductance regulator function. Pediatr Res. 2020;87:137-145. doi: 10.1038/s41390-019-0503-8.

Sato K, Sato F. Defective β-adrenergic response of cystic fibrosis sweat glands in vivo and in vitro. J Clin Invest 1984;73:1763-1771. doi: 10.1172/JCI111385.

Sato T, Vries RG, Snippert HJ, van de Wetering M, Barker N, Stange DE, van Es JH, Abo A, Kujala P, Peters PJ, Clevers H. Single Lgr5 stem cells build crypt-villus structures in vitro without a mesenchymal niche. Nature. 2009;459:262-5. doi: 10.1038/nature07935.

Sato T, Stange DE, Ferrante M, Vries RG, Van Es JH, Van den Brink S, Van Houdt WJ, Pronk A, Van Gorp J, Siersema PD, Clevers H. Long-term expansion of epithelial organoids from human colon, adenoma, adenocarcinoma, and Barrett's epithelium. Gastroenterology. 2011;141:1762-72. doi: 10.1053/j.gastro.2011.07.050.

Schjoldager KT, Narimatsu Y, Joshi HJ, Clausen H. Global view of human protein glycosylation pathways and functions. Nat Rev Mol Cell Biol. 2020;21:729-749. doi: 10.1038/s41580-020-00294-x.

Schucht S, Minso R, Lex C, Reiss J, Stanke F, Tamm S, van Barneveld A, Tümmler B. Functional analysis of the p.[Arg74Trp;Val201Met;Asp1270Asn]/p.Phe508del CFTR mutation genotype in human native colon. Mol Genet Genomic Med. 2019;7:e00526. doi: 10.1002/mgg3.526.

Schutgens F, Rookmaaker MB, Margaritis T, Rios A, Ammerlaan C, Jansen J, Gijzen L, Vormann M, Vonk A, Viveen M, Yengej FY, Derakhshan S, de Winter-de Groot KM, Artegiani B, van Boxtel R, Cuppen E, Hendrickx APA, van den Heuvel-Eibrink MM, Heitzer E, Lanz H, Beekman J, Murk JL, Masereeuw R, Holstege F, Drost J, Verhaar MC, Clevers H. Tubuloids derived from human adult kidney and urine for personalized disease modeling. Nat Biotechnol. 2019;37:303-313. doi: 10.1038/s41587-019-0048-8.

Schwank G, Koo BK, Sasselli V, Dekkers JF, Heo I, Demircan T, Sasaki N, Boymans S, Cuppen E, van der Ent CK, Nieuwenhuis EE, Beekman JM, Clevers H. Functional repair of CFTR by CRISPR/Cas9 in intestinal stem cell organoids of cystic fibrosis patients. Cell Stem Cell. 2013;13:653-8. doi: 10.1016/j.stem.2013.11.002.

Sermet-Gaudelus I, Vallée B, Urbin I, Torossi T, Marianovski R, Fajac A, Feuillet MN, Bresson JL, Lenoir G, Bernaudin JF, Edelman A. Normal function of the cystic fibrosis conductance regulator protein can be associated with homozygous ΔF508 mutation. Pediatr Res. 2002; 52:628-35. doi: 10.1203/00006450-200211000-00005.

Sermet-Gaudelus I, Girodon E, Sands D, Stremmler N, Vavrova V, Deneuville E, Reix P, Bui S, Huet F, Lebourgeois M, Munck A, Iron A, Skalicka V, Bienvenu T, Roussel D, Lenoir G, Bellon G, Sarles J, Macek M, Roussey M, Fajac I, Edelman A. Clinical phenotype and genotype of children with borderline sweat test and abnormal nasal epithelial chloride transport. Am J Respir Crit Care Med. 2010;182:929-36. doi: 10.1164/rccm.201003-0382OC.

Sermet-Gaudelus I, Nguyen-Khoa T, Hatton A, Hayes K, Pranke I. Sweat chloride testing and nasal potential difference (NPD) are primary outcome parameters in treatment with Cystic Fibrosis Transmembrane Conductance Regulator (CFTR) modulators. J Pers Med. 2021; 11:729. doi: 10.3390/jpm11080729.

Solomon GM, Konstan MW, Wilschanski M, Billings J, Sermet-Gaudelus I, Accurso F, Vermeulen F, Levin E, Hathorne H, Reeves G, Sabbatini G, Hill A, Mayer-Hamblett N, Ashlock M, Clancy JP, Rowe SM. An international randomized multicenter comparison of nasal potential difference techniques. Chest 2010;138:919-28. doi: 10.1378/chest.10-0179.

Sommerburg O, Lindner M, Muckenthaler M, Kohlmueller D, Leible S, Feneberg R, Kulozik AE, Mall MA, Hoffmann GF. Initial evaluation of a biochemical cystic fibrosis newborn screening by sequential analysis of immunoreactive trypsinogen and pancreatitis-associated protein (IRT/PAP) as a strategy that does not involve DNA testing in a Northern European population. J Inherit Metab Dis. 2010;33(Suppl 2):S263-71. doi: 10.1007/s10545-010-9174-7.

Sousa M, Servidoni MF, Vinagre AM, Ramalho AS, Bonadia LC, Felício V, Ribeiro MA, Uliyakina I, Marson FA, Kmit A, Cardoso SR, Ribeiro JD, Bertuzzo CS, Sousa L, Kunzelmann K, Ribeiro AF, Amaral MD. Measurements of CFTR-mediated Cl- secretion in human rectal biopsies constitute a robust biomarker for Cystic Fibrosis diagnosis and prognosis. PLoS One. 2012;7:e47708. doi: 10.1371/journal.pone.0047708.

Standaert TA, Boitano L, Emerson J, Milgram LJ, Konstan MW, Hunter J, Berclaz PY, Brass L, Zeitlin PL, Hammond K, Davies Z, Foy C, Noone PG, Knowles MR. Standardized procedure for measurement of nasal potential difference: an outcome measure in multicenter cystic fibrosis clinical trials. Pediatr Pulmonol. 2004; 37:385-92. doi: 10.1002/ppul.10448.

Stanke F, Ballmann M, Bronsveld I, Dörk T, Gallati S, Laabs U, Derichs N, Ritzka M, Posselt HG, Harms HK, Griese M, Blau H, Mastella G, Bijman J, Veeze H, Tümmler B. Diversity of the basic defect of homozygous *CFTR* mutation genotypes in humans. J Med Genet. 2008; 45:47-54. doi: 10.1136/jmg.2007.053561.

Stanke F, van Barneveld A, Hedtfeld S, Wölfl S, Becker T, Tümmler B. The CF-modifying gene EHF promotes p.Phe508del-CFTR residual function by altering protein glycosylation and trafficking in epithelial cells. Eur J Hum Genet. 2014;22:660-6. doi: 10.1038/ejhg.2013.209.

Sun X, Yi Y, Yan Z, Rosen BH, Liang B, Winter MC, Evans TIA, Rotti PG, Yang Y, Gray JS, Park SY, Zhou W, Zhang Y, Moll SR, Woody L, Tran DM, Jiang L, Vonk AM, Beekman JM, Negulescu P, Van Goor F, Fiorino DF, Gibson-Corley KN, Engelhardt JF. In utero and postnatal VX-770 administration rescues multiorgan disease in a ferret model of cystic fibrosis. Sci Transl Med. 2019; 11:eaau7531. doi: 10.1126/scitranslmed.aau7531.

Treggiari D, Kleinfelder K, Bertini M, Tridello G, Fedrigo A, Pintani E, Iansa P, Casiraghi A, Minghetti P, Cipolli M, Sorio C, Melotti P. Optical measurements of sweat for in vivo quantification of CFTR function in individual sweat glands. J Cyst Fibros. 2021;20:824-827. doi: 10.1016/j.jcf.2021.03.003.

van Barneveld A, Stanke F, Tamm S, Siebert B, Brandes G, Derichs N, Ballmann M, Junge S, Tümmler B. Functional analysis of F508del CFTR in native human colon. Biochim Biophys Acta. 2010;1802:1062-9. doi: 10.1016/j.bbadis.2010.08.001.

van Barneveld A, Stanke F, Claass A, Ballmann M, Tümmler B. CFTR protein analysis of splice site mutation 2789+5 G-A. J Cyst Fibros. 2008;7:165-7. doi: 10.1016/j.jcf.2007.07.007.

Veeze HJ, Sinaasappel M, Bijman J, Bouquet J, De Jonge HR. Ion transport abnormalities in rectal suction biopsies from childern with cystic fibrosis. Gastroenterology 1991;101:398-403. doi: 10.1016/0016-5085(91)90017-f

Veeze HJ, Halley DJ, Bijman J, de Jongste JC, de Jonge HR, Sinaasappel M. Determinants of mild clinical symptoms in cystic fibrosis patients. Residual chloride secretion measured in rectal biopsies in relation to the genotype. J Clin Invest. 1994;93:461-6. doi: 10.1172/JCI116993.

Verstegen MMA, Roos FJM, Burka K, Gehart H, Jager M, de Wolf M, Bijvelds MJC, de Jonge HR, Ardisasmita AI, van Huizen NA, Roest HP, de Jonge J, Koch M, Pampaloni F, Fuchs SA, Schene IF, Luider TM, van der Doef HPJ, Bodewes FAJA, de Kleine RHJ, Spee B, Kremers GJ, Clevers H, IJzermans JNM, Cuppen E, van der Laan LJW. Human extrahepatic and intrahepatic cholangiocyte organoids show region-specific differentiation potential and model cystic fibrosis-related bile duct disease. Sci Rep. 2020;10:21900. doi: 10.1038/s41598-020-79082-8.

Wilschanski M, Famini H, Strauss-Liviatan N, Rivlin J, Blau H, Bibi H, Bentur L, Yahav Y, Springer H, Kramer MR, Klar A, Ilani A, Kerem B, Kerem E. Nasal potential difference measurements in patients with atypical cystic fibrosis. Eur Respir J. 2001;17:1208-15. doi: 10.1183/09031936.01.00092501.

Wilschanski M, Dupuis A, Ellis L, Jarvi K, Zielenski J, Tullis E, Martin S, Corey M, Tsui LC, Durie P. Mutations in the cystic fibrosis transmembrane regulator gene and in vivo transepithelial potentials. Am J Respir Crit Care Med. 2006;174:787-94. doi: 10.1164/rccm.200509-1377OC.

Yoo JS, Moyer BD, Bannykh S, Yoo HM, Riordan JR, Balch WE. Non-conventional trafficking of the cystic fibrosis transmembrane conductance regulator through the early secretory pathway. J Biol Chem 2002;277: 11401-11409. doi: 10.1074/jbc.M110263200.

Zomer-van Ommen DD, de Poel E, Kruisselbrink E, Oppelaar H, Vonk AM, Janssens HM, van der Ent CK, Hagemeijer MC, Beekman JM. Comparison of ex vivo and in vitro intestinal cystic fibrosis models to measure CFTR-dependent ion channel activity. J Cyst Fibros. 2018;17:316-324. doi: 10.1016/j.jcf.2018.02.007.

3. Endpoints of phase II and phase III trials with CFTR modulators

3.1. Lung function

Mirjam Stahl

Cystic fibrosis (CF) lung disease has the greatest impact on the quality and expectancy of life of affected patients. Although the lungs of patients with CF are structurally normal at birth, morphological abnormalities occur early in life as demonstrated by the examination of CF newborn screening cohorts using imaging techniques (Sturgess and Imrie, 1982; Sly et al., 2009). Initially only visible by subtle ventilation inhomogeneity detectable by multiple-breath washout (MBW), the abnormalities subsequently lead to reduced flows in the peripheral airways followed by pseudo-restriction due to the reduction in the forced vital capacity (FVC) and ultimately merge into reduced flows and volumes in the central airways as indicated by reduced forced expiratory volume in the first second (FEV1) detectable by spirometry (☞ Table 3.1). MBW is a useful component for recording early lung changes in newborns, infants and preschool children with CF (Stahl et al., 2014) because it is more sensitive than spirometry to detect early deficits in lung function. Likewise, MBW can unravel on-going changes such as bronchiectasis in patients with CF who present with a spirometry in the normal range (Gustafsson et al., 2008).

CF lungs are normal at birth, but postnatally ventilation becomes inhomogeneous. This ventilation inhomogeneity (VI) starts in the small airways at the onset of the disease. In contrast to the large central airways, the lung periphery down to the smallest airways is a system with low total airway resistance. Despite their share of 97% of the lung volume, the small peripheral airways beyond the 8th to 10th generation of division only contribute 15% to resistance (Macklem et al., 1967). Here gas transport mainly takes place by convection and diffusion (Robinson et al., 2009). Standard methods of lung function such as body plethysmography or spirometry are based on changes in resistance and are therefore not sensitive enough to detect pathologies in the small peripheral airways. Using MBW, the VI is determined by measuring the ventilation efficiency of a marker gas in tidal breathing. In case of nitrogen (N_2)-MBW, the inhalation is switched from room air to 100% oxygen, and the concentration of the indicator gas (N_2) is then monitored until it has fallen to 1/40 of its initial end-tidal concentration (Robinson et al., 2009; 2013; 2018). Tidal volumes, functional residual capacity (FRC_{MBW}) and the lung clearance index (LCI) as a global marker of VI are derived from the gas concentrations in the exhaled air (☞ Table 3.1).

The LCI is elevated in newborns and infants with CF shortly after birth compared to healthy controls (Gustafsson et al., 2003; Aurora et al., 2005; Owens et al., 2011). In preschool age, more children with CF had abnormal LCI than abnormal spirometry findings, with an elevated LCI in preschool age predicting both abnormal LCI and worsened spirometry (FEV1) in school age (Aurora et al., 2011; Hardaker et al., 2019; Stanojevic et al., 2021). Long-term follow-up showed that the LCI in-

Technique	Main Outcome Parameter	Applicable Age Range	Advantages	Disadvantages
Spirometry	Forced expiratory volume in 1 second (FEV1)	≥3 years	• good availability	• necessitates cooperation • insensitive to mild changes
MBW	Lung clearance index (LCI)	from infancy on (requiring sedation in some young patients)	• performed in tidal breathing with minimal cooperation • detects early ventilation inhomogeneities	• only available at specialized centers • harmonization between devices, tracer gases and protocols pending

Table 3.1: Comparison of lung function techniques used as endpoints in CFTR modulator studies.

creases over time in children and adolescents with CF (Frauchiger et al., 2020). There is a concordance between the LCI and structural and/or functional abnormalities in lung imaging (Owens et al., 2011; Hall et al., 2011; Ramsey et al., 2016; Stahl et al., 2017). Furthermore, multicenter validation and feasibility of MBW were demonstrated for several pediatric age groups (Stahl et al., 2018; 2020; Saunders et al., 2019). Thus, the LCI has been employed as an endpoint in randomized placebo-controlled double-blind phase 3 trials to test the effectiveness of mucolytic inhalations (Stahl et al., 2019) and CFTR modulators (Davies et al., 2013; Milla et al., 2017; Ratjen et al., 2017) in infants, preschoolers and young school children. Monotherapy with ivacaftor or combination therapy with ivacaftor-lumacaftor (☞ Chapter 5.3.) consistently led to a reduction of VI as indicated by a reduction of the LCI (☞ Figure 3.1).

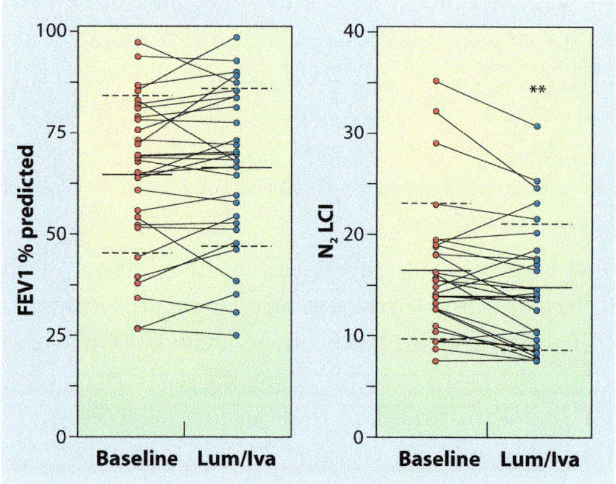

Figure 3.1: Effects of lumacaftor–ivacaftor (Lum/Iva) therapy on percentage predicted forced expiratory volume in 1 second (FEV1% predicted) and lung clearance index (LCI) in p.Phe508del homozygous patients with cystic fibrosis (Graeber et al., 2021). Paired measurements of FEV1% predicted (left panel; n=30) and LCI determined by nitrogen (N_2) multiple breath washout (right panel; n=28) at baseline and after initiation of Lum/Iva therapy. The solid lines represent the group mean, and the dashed lines represent the standard deviation of the mean. Adapted with permission of the American Thoracic Society from Graeber et al., 2021. Copyright © 2021 American Thoracic Society. All rights reserved.

In patients aged 12 years and older the LCI has so far only been used as an endpoint in a single phase IV observational study (Graeber et al., 2021). In all phase III and phase IV studies the treatment response was either only detectable or at least clearer in LCI than in FEV1 (Milla et al., 2017; Ratjen et al., 2017; Graeber et al., 2021). A recent study on the efficacy of the triple combination therapy with elexacaftor, tezacaftor and ivacaftor in school-aged CF children with at least one p.Phe508del allele revealed a strong improvement in LCI under this CFTR modulating therapy compared to the Placebo arm (☞ Figure 3.2; Zemanick et al., 2021).

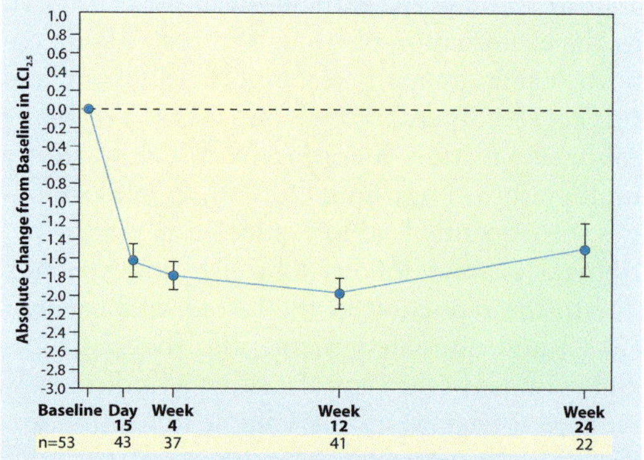

Figure 3.2: A phase 3 open-label study of elexacaftor/tezacaftor/ivacaftor in children 6 through 11 years of age with cystic fibrosis and at least one p.Phe508del allele (Zemanick et al., 2021): Absolute change from baseline at each visit in lung clearance index2.5 (LCI2.5). Adapted with permission of the American Thoracic Society from Zemanick et al., 2021. Copyright © 2021 American Thoracic Society. All rights reserved.

3.2. Imaging

Till Frederik Kaireit, Burkhard Tümmler and Jens Vogel-Claussen

Clinical studies in CF, particularly in the field of CFTR modulators, have commonly used spirometry (FEV1) and anthropometry (weight, BMI) as primary and secondary endpoints. CF clinics routinely apply imaging techniques such as chest roentgenograms and abdomen ultrasound to monitor the course of the individual patient, but chest imaging as a surrogate parameter for efficacy in clinical trials has just recently received momentum.

Conventional frontal/lateral chest radiographs and the corresponding Chrispin-Norman, Brasfield and Wisconsin scoring systems (Chrispin and Norman, 1974; Brasfield et al., 1979; Weatherly et al., 1993) lack the needed sensitivity to resolve the short-term changes within the time frame of a clinical trial, particularly in subjects with advanced lung disease, albeit substantial progress has been made to improve among-observer agreement (Cleveland et al., 2014) and automatic scoring by machine-learning techniques (Zucker et al., 2020).

High-resolution chest computed tomography (CT) is a highly sensitive technique to reliably visualize the morphological abnormalities of CF lung disease, i.e. mucus plugging with distal atelectasis, bronchial wall thickening, air-trapping, sacculations, bullae, solid and ground-glass opacities, and central and upper lobe predominant bronchiectasis (Crowley et al., 2021). Multiple scoring systems such as CF-CT (Wainwright et al., 2011) or PRAGMA-CF (Rosenow et al., 2015) have been described and validated over the last 20 years, and all correlate with pulmonary exacerbation or progression of CF lung disease based on FEV1 (Goralski et al., 2021). CT has been used to examine therapeutic interventions in randomized clinical trials such as the read-through agent ataluren for CF patients carrying a nonsense mutation (☞ Chapter 4.; Kerem et al., 2014). According to the initial image analysis of CT scans by Brody II scores (Brody et al., 2004) the study participants did not show any change in their structural CF lung disease (Kerem et al., 2014), but the subsequent re-analysis of the same datasets with the more sensitive PRAGMA-CF score revealed significant increase in severity of structural lung disease during the study period (Tiddens et al., 2020). This example demonstrates the still unmet need of sensitive and standardized consensus protocols to include CT outcome measures in the assessment of response-to-treatment in randomized controlled trials.

The main limitation of the use of CT for the regular monitoring of people with CF is the cumulative radiation dose. While the effective dose of a conventional chest CT is about 5.4 mSv, a volumetric ultra-low-dose CT thorax protocol based on iterative image reconstruction algorithms has recently been developed, which results in diagnostic quality CT images at a dose of 0.08 mSv similar to that of a chest radiograph (Moloney et al., 2021). Improvement in ultra-low-dose CT imaging scores were observed after treatment with the CFTR modulators ivacaftor (Ronan et al., 2018) and elexacaftor/tezacaftor/ivacaftor (Crowley et al., 2021).

Despite this impressive amelioration, we should minimize the accumulating radiation exposure in our CF patient population who can envisage an increased lifespan with highly effective CFTR modulators. Magnetic resonance imaging (MRI) has the advantage of imaging without ionizing radiation exposure. Clinical use of MRI of the lungs has been hampered in the past by the intrinsically low MR signal caused by the low density of protons in the lungs and the rapid decay of the MR signal due to susceptibility inhomogeneity as well as respiratory and cardiac motion. These intrinsic limitations have meanwhile been overcome by advances in hard- and software.

MRI provides information about pulmonary morphology and generates quantitative data of ventilation, perfusion and gas exchange. In proton MRI, lung morphology is assessed by gradient-echo and spin-echo pulse sequences. Imaging of the passage of an intravenously given bolus of a gadolinium salt that shortens the T1 relaxation time, visualizes the pulmonary vascular system. In analogy to the CT score (Brody et al., 2004), a global MRI score was developed that consists of a perfusion score and morphological subscores for bronchial wall thickening, bronchiectasis, mucus plugging, sacculations and abscesses, consolidations, and pleural reaction (Eichinger et al., 2012; Wielpütz et al., 2014). The MRI score has been applied as outcome measure for clinical trials on the efficacy of hypersaline inhalation in CF infants (Stahl et al., 2019) and of lumacaftor/ivacaftor in CF preschoolers, the worldwide first randomized, double-blind, placebo-controlled drug intervention study in this age group.

Meanwhile lung proton MRI made further progress, namely ultra-short echo time MRI, oxygen enhanced MRI, Fourier decomposition MRI and other related methods including self-gated non-contrast-enhanced functional lung MRI and phase-resolved functional lung imaging (☞ the review by Voskrebenzev and Vogel-Claussen [2021] for further details). For example, ultra-short echo time MRI has dramatically improved the signal-to-noise ratio and the spatial resolution of lung MRI compatible with CT (Dournes et al., 2016). For Fourier decomposition MRI, a conventional steady-state free precession sequence optimized to gain high temporal resolution is used to acquire a time series of images. In post-processing, signal

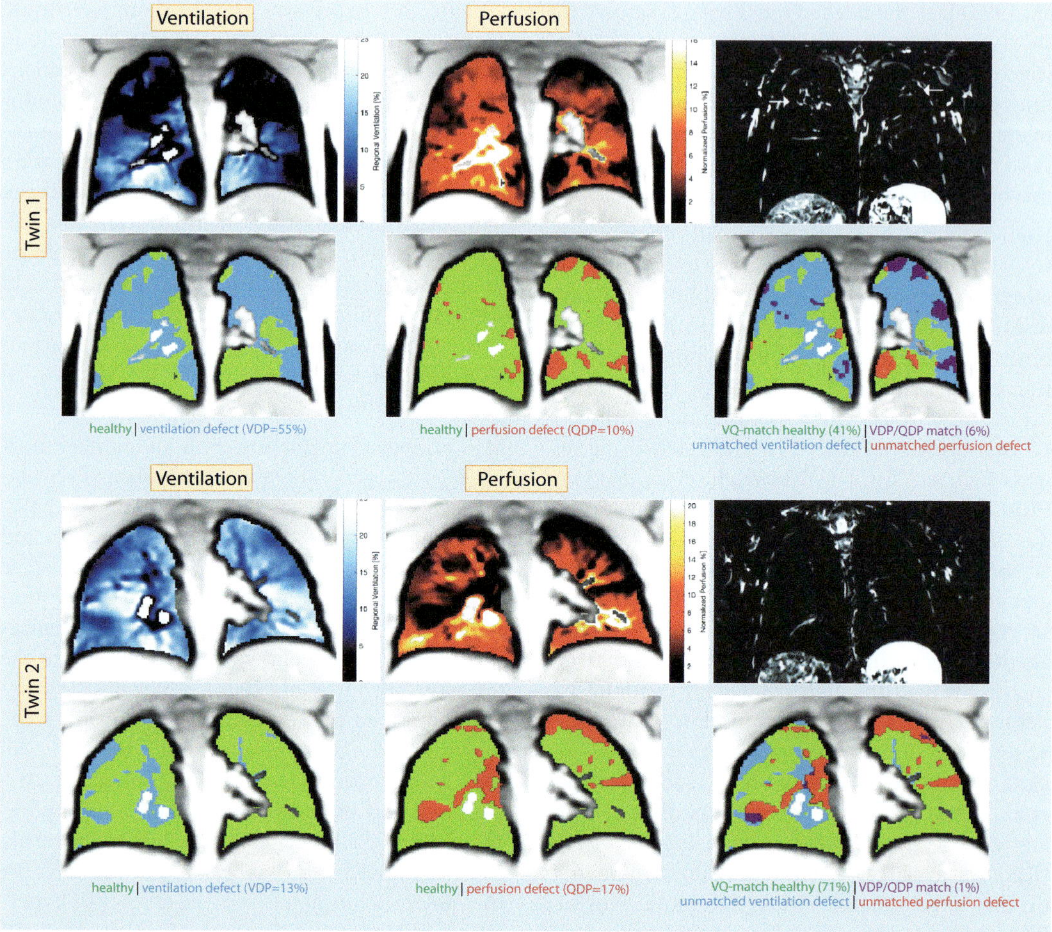

Figure 3.3: **Phase resolved functional lung (PREFUL) MRI in 26-year-old monozygous CF twins.** Tidal breathing was captured with coronal slices using a standard spoiled gradient echo sequence with high temporal resolution of ~3 images/s requiring 1 min/slice on a 1.5 T scanner. The resulting time series were further analyzed by the automated post-processing pipeline PREFUL (Voskrebenzev et al., 2018), which ultimately results in segmented ventilation and perfusion maps. During post-processing, images were sorted by their cardiac phase and registered to an intermediate lung position or further sorted by their respiratory state (i.e., retrospective gating resulting in a higher temporal resolution). Applying a Fourier transform allows to separate signal changes caused by ventilation from those caused by perfusion.

To generate ventilation maps, signal changes between two inflation states during tidal breathing (end-inspiration and end-expiration) were compared. A stochastically driven threshold was applied to each individual slice to create defect maps and calculate a ventilation defect percentage (VDP). The averaged aorta signal of the coronal slice at the middle of the tracheal level and average heart frequency of the respective acquisition were used to quantify perfusion (Q) in mL/min/100 mL according to Kjørstad et al. (2014) followed by threshold based calculation of a perfusion defect percentage (QDP).

Exemplary coronal PREFUL MRI-derived regional ventilation (left column) and perfusion-weighted images (middle column) with ventilation defect percentage (VDP, blue), perfusion defect percentage (QDP, red) and ventilation/perfusion (VDP/QDP) maps (purple signifying matched ventilation-perfusion-defects and green matched healthy parenchyma) are shown. Twin 1 (160 cm, 50 kg, BMI 19.5 kg/m², FEV1 28% predicted, LCI 20.0) has typical heterogeneous areas of hypoventilation (blue) and hypoperfusion (red) mainly because of mucus plugging and bronchial wall thickening in the central upper airways (white arrows), as shown on the corresponding turbo inversion magnitude image. These defects are partly matched on the VDP/QDP map (purple). Twin 2 (160 cm, 60 kg, BMI 23.4 kg/m², FEV1 86% predicted, LCI 15.3) shows less mucus plugging and bronchial wall thickening resulting in lower VDP and QDP values, but also small heterogeneous areas of hypoventilation (blue) and hypoperfusion (red).

modulations caused by respiratory and cardiac motion are separated by their frequencies so that maps of ventilation and perfusion can be generated (Bauman et al., 2009). The related method of phase sorting according to cardiac and ventilation phases generates phase-resolved functional lung (PREFUL) perfusion and ventilation cycles with increased temporal resolution (Voskrebenzev et al., 2018). Moreover, perfusion-weighted PREFUL MRI automatically calculates the regional pulmonary perfusion impairment in CF patients (Behrendt et al., 2020). All these novel methods offer a regional free-breathing test without any contrast agent and are predestined for application in young children. Figure 3.3 shows an instructive application of PREFUL MRI to visualize the broad variability of CF lung disease even in genetically identical monozygous CF twins.

Besides proton MRI other isotopes with a nonzero nuclear spin are used for pulmonary MRI. Inhaled hyperpolarized noble gases, ^{129}Xenon being most commonly used, increases the MRI signal by about five orders of magnitude. Imaging ^{129}Xe during a tidal inspiration allows the regional quantification of lung ventilation with high spatial resolution and high signal-to-noise ratio (Thomen et al., 2015). The high sensitivity of hyperpolarized gas ventilation-MRI was demonstrated in CF patients with very mild lung disease detecting ventilation defects in subjects with normal spirometry and LCI and no structural abnormalities in the CT scan (Marshall et al., 2017). Alternatively, fluorinated gases may be applied to map pulmonary ventilation by MRI. ^{19}F MRI imaging identifies ventilation defects and areas of differential wash-in and wash-out kinetics of the fluorinated gas (Goralski et al., 2020). The gas wash-out time constant has been shown to distinguish between healthy volunteers and patients with CF who have normal spirometry (FEV1 >80%), pointing toward its potential utility for early/mild disease (Goralski et al., 2020).

In summary, we have now a large portfolio of methods at hand to incorporate MRI lung imaging as an outcome measure into clinical trials.

3.3. Extra-pulmonary endpoints

Jochen G. Mainz

In the first trials assessing effects of ivacaftor in people with CF carrying a p.GlyG551Asp mutation (Ramsey et al., 2011), extra-pulmonary endpoints were not directly assessed except for effects on sweat glands. The primary outcome parameter in all early studies was pulmonary function assessed by changes of FEV1%predicted and, later, also changes in LCI. In these patients newly receiving ivacaftor, sweat tests (☞ Chapter 2.1.) revealed a substantial decrease from about 100 to about 50 mmol/L Cl^{-}, as also recently seen with triple modulator therapy (☞ Chapter 5.3.). However, sweat test results did not correlate with the individual's changes in pulmonary function.

Most of the unexpected extra-pulmonary effects were only captured indirectly, e.g. by substantial weight gain as well as by improvement in Quality of Life. Altogether, these effects of CFTR modulators exceeded by far the changes of pulmonary function.

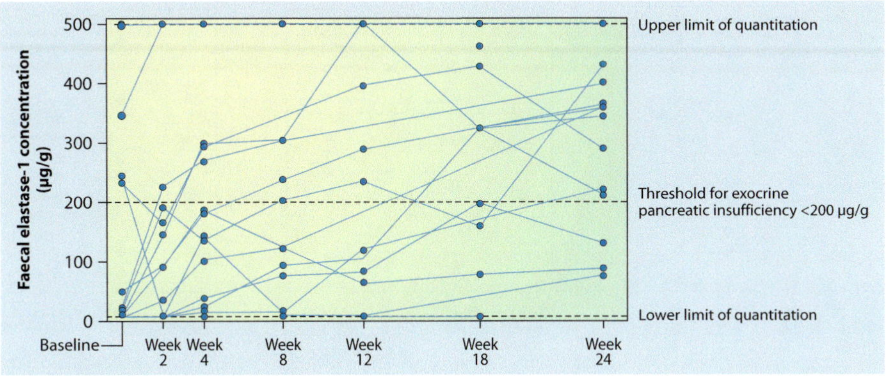

Figure 3.4: Increase of pancreatic elastase in stool in CF children aged 12-24 month carrying a gating mutation newly receiving ivacaftor (Rosenfeld et al., 2018).

Only after approval of ivacaftor in many countries, case series reported the loss of pancreatic insufficiency in some children (Mainz et al., 2018). When pancreatic elastase was included into trials on safety and effectivity of ivacaftor in children carrying a p.Gly551Asp mutation, a substantial increase of this marker of pancreatic function was found (Davies et al., 2016; ☞ Figure 3.4). Such trends were also seen in studies assessing the effects of lumacaftor/ivacaftor in children homozygous for p.Phe508del (Milla et al., 2017). However, pancreatic destruction in young children is more advanced in p.Phe508del homozygotes than in carriers of a p.Gly551Asp mutation. Accordingly, recovery of pancreatic sufficiency is not probable in the Phe508del cohort, unless potent modulator therapy is initiated during pregnancy or early infancy. Stepwise approval of other highly effective CFTR modulators like elexacaftor/tezacaftor/ivacaftor for younger children will reveal whether early administration may also modify pancreatic function in other *CFTR* genotypes.

In contrast to the 85% of CF patients with pancreatic insufficiency, the remaining 15% of patients with a milder CFTR phenotype carrying a class IV-VI mutation are typically pancreatic sufficient. Due to their remaining functional pancreatic tissue these patients are at special risk for acute and recurrent episodes of pancreatitis. Interestingly, in a case series of 6 patients with gating mutations and recurrent pancreatitis treatment with ivacaftor led to cessation of pancreatic exacerbations after a period of 6 months (Carrion et al., 2018).

In the gastro-enteric passage, CF patients tend to have a decreased pH for lacking bicarbonate secretion. Consequently, an optimal pH between 5.5 and 6, also required for optimal activation of micro-encapsulated enzyme supplements, is only reached with a considerable delay. This pathology was compensated by CFTR modulation with ivacaftor in patients carrying a gating mutation, as shown using wireless motility capsules (Gelfond et al., 2017). Furthermore, this effect will have contributed to improvement of the nutritional status of people with CF treated with potent CFTR modulators.

For identification and quantification of the multiorganic abdominal symptoms specifically designed for CF patients, the CFAbd-Score has been developed following FDA guidelines (Tabori et al., 2017a; 2017b; Jaudszus et al., 2019). Recently, we assessed changes of abdominal symptoms during the triple therapy with elexacaftor/tezacaftor/ivacaftor in Irish and British CF patients. After only one month of therapy, we found a significant decrease of 25% in the total symptoms score which comprises 28 items. Future longitudinal studies of triple therapy will implement the CFAbd-Score and assess changes in markers of abdominal inflammation including faecal calprotectin.

Effects of CFTR modulators on intestinal mucosa can also be quantified ex vivo assessing intestinal current measurements (ICM) from rectal biopsies mounted in micro-Ussing chambers (Graeber et al., 2015; 2018; ☞ Chapter 2.3.). Similarly, CFTR-mediated chloride conductance of the upper respi-

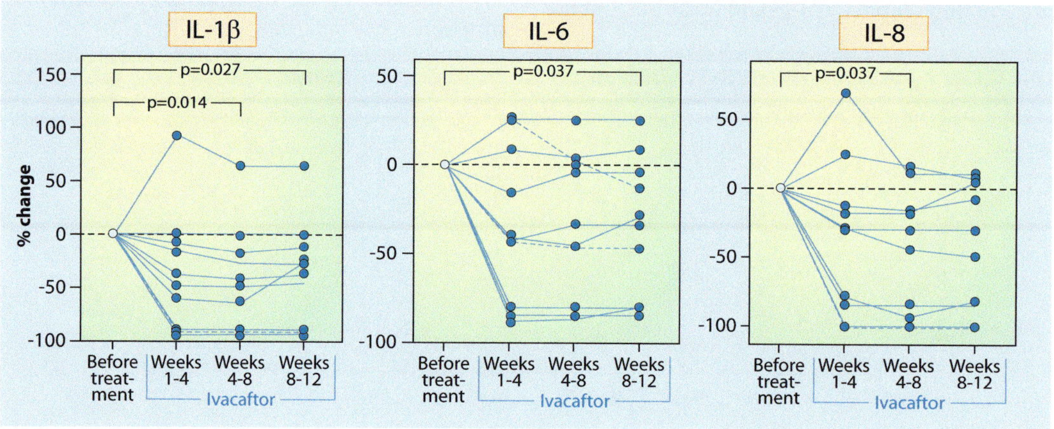

Figure 3.5: Cumulative changes of inflammatory cytokines compared to baseline in nasal lavage from CF patients with a p.Gly551Asp allele who started the treatment with ivacaftor (Mainz et al., 2021).

ratory epithelium can be assessed by nasal potential difference measurements (Graeber et al., 2018; ☞ Chapter 2.2.).

Clinical effects in the sinonasal compartment of new therapy with ivacaftor (Davies et al., 2013) had been identified as unexpected events including symptoms of rhinosinusitis. Primarily discussed as a side effect, these symptoms in fact represent the mobilization of secretions and crusts and are the first signs of recovery. In the long run, CFTR-function was re-established in the sinonasal compartment. Upper airway symptoms assessed with the SNOT20 score decreased (McCormick et al., 2019) and, over many months, a substantial improvement of rhinosinusitis was evident in sinonasal CT scans, including reduction of polyps (Sheikh et al., 2015). Moreover, inflammation of the sinonasal compartment decreased as indicated by the reduction of inflammatory mediators in serially taken nasal lavages (☞ Figure 3.5; Mainz et al., 2021).

In conclusion, extra-pulmonary endpoints should be part of any trial that examines the clinical efficacy of CFTR modulator therapy.

3.4. References

Aurora P, Bush A, Gustafsson P, Oliver C, Wallis C, Price J, Stroobant J, Carr S, Stocks J; London Cystic Fibrosis Collaboration. Multiple-breath washout as a marker of lung disease in preschool children with cystic fibrosis. Am J Respir Crit Care Med. 2005;171:249-56. doi: 10.1164/rccm.200407-895OC.

Aurora P, Stanojevic S, Wade A, Oliver C, Kozlowska W, Lum S, Bush A, Price J, Carr SB, Shankar A, Stocks J; London Cystic Fibrosis Collaboration. Lung clearance index at 4 years predicts subsequent lung function in children with cystic fibrosis. Am J Respir Crit Care Med. 2011; 183:752-8. doi:10.1164/rccm.200911-1646OC.

Bauman G, Puderbach M, Deimling M, Jellus V, Chefd' hotel C, Dinkel J, Hintze C, Kauczor HU, Schad LR. Non-contrast-enhanced perfusion and ventilation assessment of the human lung by means of fourier decomposition in proton MRI. Magn Reson Med. 2009;62:656-64. doi: 10.1002/mrm.22031.

Behrendt L, Voskrebenzev A, Klimeš F, Gutberlet M, Winther HB, Kaireit TF, Alsady TM, Pöhler GH, Derlin T, Wacker F, Vogel-Claussen J. Validation of automated Perfusion-Weighted Phase-Resolved Functional Lung (PREFUL)-MRI in patients with pulmonary diseases. J Magn Reson Imaging. 2020;52:103-114. doi: 10.1002/jmri.27027.

Brasfield D, Hicks G, Soong S, Tiller RE. The chest roentgenogram in cystic fibrosis: a new scoring system. Pediatrics. 1979;63:24-9.

Brody AS, Klein JS, Molina PL, Quan J, Bean JA, Wilmott RW. High-resolution computed tomography in young patients with cystic fibrosis: distribution of abnormalities and correlation with pulmonary function tests. J Pediatr. 2004;145:32-8. doi: 10.1016/j.jpeds.2004.02.038.

Carrion A, Borowitz DS, Freedman SD, Siracusa CM, Goralski JL, Hadjiliadis D, Srinivasan S, Stokes DC. Reduction of recurrence risk of pancreatitis in cystic fibrosis with ivacaftor: Case series. J Pediatr Gastroenterol Nutr. 2018;66:451-454. doi: 10.1097/MPG.0000000000001788.

Chrispin AR, Norman AP. The systematic evaluation of the chest radiograph in cystic fibrosis. Pediatr Radiol. 1974;2:101-5.

Cleveland RH, Stamoulis C, Sawicki G, Kelliher E, Zucker EJ, Wood C, Cleveland RH, Stamoulis C, Sawicki G, Kelliher E, Zucker EJ, Wood C, Zurakowski D, Lee E. Brasfield and Wisconsin scoring systems have equal value as outcome assessment tools of cystic fibrosis lung disease. Pediatr Radiol. 2014;44:529-34. doi: 10.1007/s00247-013-2848-1

Crowley C, Connor OJO, Ciet P, Tiddens HAWM, Maher MM. The evolving role of radiological imaging in cystic fibrosis. Curr Opin Pulm Med. 2021;27:575-585. doi: 10.1097/MCP.0000000000000828.

Davies J, Sheridan H, Bell N, Cunningham S, Davis SD, Elborn JS, Milla CE, Starner TD, Weiner DJ, Lee PS, Ratjen F. Assessment of clinical response to ivacaftor with lung clearance index in cystic fibrosis patients with a G551D-CFTR mutation and preserved spirometry: a randomised controlled trial. Lancet Respir Med. 2013;1: 630-638. doi: 10.1016/S2213-2600(13)70182-6.

Davies JC, Cunningham S, Harris WT, Lapey A, Regelmann WE, Sawicki GS, Southern KW, Robertson S, Green Y, Cooke J, Rosenfeld M; KIWI Study Group. Safety, pharmacokinetics, and pharmacodynamics of ivacaftor in patients aged 2-5 years with cystic fibrosis and a CFTR gating mutation (KIWI): an open-label, single-arm study. Lancet Respir Med. 2016;4:107-15. doi: 10.1016/S2213-2600(15)00545-7.

Dournes G, Menut F, Macey J, Fayon M, Chateil JF, Salel M, Corneloup O, Montaudon M, Berger P, Laurent F. Lung morphology assessment of cystic fibrosis using MRI with ultra-short echo time at submillimeter spatial resolution. Eur Radiol. 2016;26:3811-3820. doi: 10.1007/s00330-016-4218-5.

Eichinger M, Optazaite DE, Kopp-Schneider A, Hintze C, Biederer J, Niemann A, Mall MA, Wielpütz MO, Kauczor HU, Puderbach M. Morphologic and functional scoring of cystic fibrosis lung disease using MRI. Eur J Radiol. 2012;81:1321-9. doi: 10.1016/j.ejrad.2011.02.045.

Frauchiger BS, Binggeli S, Yammine S, Spycher B, Krüger L, Ramsey KA, Latzin P. Longitudinal course of clinical lung clearance index in children with cystic fibrosis. Eur Respir J. 2021;58:2002686. doi: 10.1183/13993003.02686-2020.

Gelfond D, Heltshe S, Ma C, Rowe SM, Frederick C, Uluer A, Sicilian L, Konstan M, Tullis E, Roach RN, Griffin K, Joseloff E, Borowitz D. Impact of CFTR modulation on intestinal pH, motility, and clinical outcomes in patients with cystic fibrosis and the G551D mutation. Clin Transl Gastroenterol. 2017;8:e81. doi: 10.1038/ctg.2017.10.

Goralski JL, Chung SH, Glass TM, Ceppe AS, Akinnagbe-Zusterzeel EO, Trimble AT, Boucher RC, Soher BJ, Charles HC, Donaldson SH, Lee YZ. Dynamic perfluorinated gas MRI reveals abnormal ventilation despite normal FEV1 in cystic fibrosis. JCI Insight. 2020;5:e133400. doi: 10.1172/jci.insight.133400.

Goralski JL, Stewart NJ, Woods JC. Novel imaging techniques for cystic fibrosis lung disease. Pediatr Pulmonol. 2021;56 Suppl 1:S40-S54. doi: 10.1002/ppul.24931.

Graeber SY, Hug MJ, Sommerburg O, Hirtz S, Hentschel J, Heinzmann A, Dopfer C, Schulz A, Mainz JG, Tümmler B, Mall MA. Intestinal current measurements detect activation of mutant CFTR in patients with cystic fibrosis with the G551D mutation treated with ivacaftor. Am J Respir Crit Care Med. 2015;192:1252-5. doi: 10.1164/rccm.201507-1271LE.

Graeber SY, Dopfer C, Naehrlich L, Gyulumyan L, Scheuermann H, Hirtz S, Wege S, Mairbäurl H, Dorda M, Hyde R, Bagheri-Hanson A, Rueckes-Nilges C, Fischer S, Mall MA, Tümmler B. Effects of lumacaftor-ivacaftor therapy on cystic fibrosis transmembrane conductance regulator function in Phe508del homozygous patients with cystic fibrosis. Am J Respir Crit Care Med. 2018;197:1433-1442. doi: 10.1164/rccm.201710-1983OC.

Graeber SY, Boutin S, Wielpütz MO, Joachim C, Frey DL, Wege S, Sommerburg O, Kauczor HU, Stahl M, Dalpke AH, Mall MA. Effects of lumacaftor-ivacaftor on lung clearance index, magnetic resonance imaging, and airway microbiome in Phe508del homozygous patients with cystic fibrosis. Ann Am Thorac Soc. 2021;18:971-980. doi: 10.1513/AnnalsATS.202008-1054OC.

Gustafsson PM, Aurora P, Lindblad A. Evaluation of ventilation maldistribution as an early indicator of lung disease in children with cystic fibrosis. Eur Respir J. 2003;22:972-9. doi: 10.1183/09031936.03.00049502.

Gustafsson PM, De Jong PA, Tiddens HA, Lindblad A. Multiple-breath inert gas washout and spirometry versus structural lung disease in cystic fibrosis. Thorax. 2008;63:129-34. doi: 10.1136/thx.2007.077784.

Hall GL, Logie KM, Parsons F, Schulzke SM, Nolan G, Murray C, Ranganathan S, Robinson P, Sly PD, Stick SM; AREST CF, Berry L, Garratt L, Massie J, Mott L, Poreddy S, Simpson S. Air trapping on chest CT is associated with worse ventilation distribution in infants with cystic fibrosis diagnosed following newborn screening. PLoS One. 2011;6:e23932. doi: 10.1371/journal.pone.0023932.

Hardaker KM, Panda H, Hulme K, Wong A, Coward E, Cooper P, Fitzgerald DA, Pandit C, Towns S, Selvadurai H, Robinson PD. Abnormal preschool Lung Clearance Index (LCI) reflects clinical status and predicts lower spirometry later in childhood in cystic fibrosis. J Cyst Fibros. 2019;18:721-727. doi: 10.1016/j.jcf.2019.02.007.

Jaudszus A, Zeman E, Jans T, Pfeifer E, Tabori H, Arnold C, Michl RK, Lorenz M, Beiersdorf N, Mainz JG. Validity and reliability of a novel multimodal questionnaire for the assessment of abdominal symptoms in people with cystic fibrosis (CFAbd-Score). Patient. 2019;12:419-428. doi: 10.1007/s40271-019-00361-2.

Kerem E, Konstan MW, De Boeck K, Accurso FJ, Sermet-Gaudelus I, Wilschanski M, Elborn JS, Melotti P, Bronsveld I, Fajac I, Malfroot A, Rosenbluth DB, Walker PA, McColley SA, Knoop C, Quattrucci S, Rietschel E, Zeitlin PL, Barth J, Elfring GL, Welch EM, Branstrom A, Spiegel RJ, Peltz SW, Ajayi T, Rowe SM; Cystic Fibrosis Ataluren Study Group. Ataluren for the treatment of nonsense-mutation cystic fibrosis: a randomised, double-blind, placebo-controlled phase 3 trial. Lancet Respir Med. 2014;2:539-47. doi: 10.1016/S2213-2600(14)70100-6.

Kjørstad Å, Corteville DM, Fischer A, Henzler T, Schmid-Bindert G, Zöllner FG, Schad LR. Quantitative lung perfusion evaluation using Fourier decomposition perfusion MRI. Magn Reson Med. 2014;72:558-62. doi: 10.1002/mrm.24930.

Macklem PT, Mead J. Resistance of central and peripheral airways measured by a retrograde catheter. J Appl Physiol. 1967;22:395-401. doi: 10.1152/jappl.1967.22.3.395.

Mainz JG, Arnold C, Hentschel J, Tabori H. Effects of ivacaftor in three pediatric siblings with cystic fibrosis carrying the mutations G551D and F508del. Arch Bronconeumol (Engl Ed). 2018;54:232-234. doi: 10.1016/j.arbres.2017.09.012.

Mainz JG, Arnold C, Wittstock K, Hipler UC, Lehmann T, Zagoya C, Duckstein F, Ellemunter H, Hentschel J. Ivacaftor reduces inflammatory mediators in upper airway lining fluid from cystic fibrosis patients with a G551D mutation: Serial non-invasive home-based collection of upper airway lining fluid. Front Immunol. 2021;12:642180. doi: 10.3389/fimmu.2021.642180.

Marshall H, Horsley A, Taylor CJ, Smith L, Hughes D, Horn FC, Swift AJ, Parra-Robles J, Hughes PJ, Norquay G, Stewart NJ, Collier GJ, Teare D, Cunningham S, Aldag I, Wild JM. Detection of early subclinical lung disease in children with cystic fibrosis by lung ventilation imaging with hyperpolarized gas MRI. Thorax. 2017;72:760-762. doi: 10.1136/thoraxjnl-2016-208948.

McCormick J, Cho DY, Lampkin B, Richman J, Hathorne H, Rowe SM, Woodworth BA. Ivacaftor improves rhinologic, psychologic, and sleep-related quality of life in G551D cystic fibrosis patients. Int Forum Allergy Rhinol. 2019;9:292-297.doi: 10.1002/alr.22251.

Milla CE, Ratjen F, Marigowda G, Liu F, Waltz D, Rosenfeld M; VX13-809-011 Part B Investigator Group. Lumacaftor/Ivacaftor in patients aged 6-11 years with cystic fibrosis and homozygous for F508del-CFTR. Am J Respir Crit Care Med. 2017;195:912-920. doi: 10.1164/rccm.201608-1754OC.

Moloney F, Kavanagh RG, Ronan NJ, Grey TM, Joyce S, Ryan DJ, Moore N, O'Connor OJ, Plant BJ, Maher MM. Ultra-low-dose thoracic CT with model-based iterative reconstruction (MBIR) in cystic fibrosis patients undergoing treatment with cystic fibrosis transmembrane conductance regulators (CFTR). Clin Radiol. 2021;76:393.e9-393.e17. doi: 10.1016/j.crad.2020.12.003.

Owens CM, Aurora P, Stanojevic S, Bush A, Wade A, Oliver C, Calder A, Price J, Carr SB, Shankar A, Stocks J; London Cystic Fibrosis Collaboration. Lung Clearance Index and HRCT are complementary markers of lung abnormalities in young children with CF. Thorax. 2011; 66:481-8. doi:10.1136/thx.2010.150375.

Ramsey BW, Davies J, McElvaney NG, Tullis E, Bell SC, Drevinek P, Griese M, McKone EF, Wainwright CE, Konstan MW, Moss R, Ratjen F, Sermet-Gaudelus I, Rowe SM, Dong Q, Rodriguez S, Yen K, Ordoñez C, Elborn JS; VX08-770-102 Study Group. A CFTR potentiator in patients with cystic fibrosis and the G551D mutation. N Engl J Med. 2011;365:1663-72. doi: 10.1056/NEJMoa1105185.

Ramsey KA, Rosenow T, Turkovic L, Skoric B, Banton G, Adams AM, Simpson SJ, Murray C, Ranganathan SC, Stick SM, Hall GL; AREST CF. Lung clearance index and structural lung disease on computed tomography in early cystic fibrosis. Am J Respir Crit Care Med. 2016; 193:60-7. doi: 10.1164/rccm.201507-1409OC.

Ratjen F, Hug C, Marigowda G, Tian S, Huang X, Stanojevic S, Milla CE, Robinson PD, Waltz D, Davies JC; VX14-809-109 investigator group. Efficacy and safety of lumacaftor and ivacaftor in patients aged 6-11 years with cystic fibrosis homozygous for F508del-CFTR: a randomised, placebo-controlled phase 3 trial. Lancet Respir Med. 2017;5:557-567. doi: 10.1016/S2213-2600(17)30215-1.

Robinson PD, Goldman MD, Gustafsson PM. Inert gas washout: theoretical background and clinical utility in respiratory disease. Respiration. 2009;78:339-55. doi: 10.1159/000225373.

Robinson PD, Latzin P, Verbanck S, Hall GL, Horsley A, Gappa M, Thamrin C, Arets HG, Aurora P, Fuchs SI, King GG, Lum S, Macleod K, Paiva M, Pillow JJ, Ranganathan S, Ratjen F, Singer F, Sonnappa S, Stocks J, Subbarao P, Thompson BR, Gustafsson PM. Consensus statement for inert gas washout measurement using multiple- and single- breath tests. Eur Respir J. 2013; 41:507-22. doi:10.1183/09031936.00069712.

Robinson PD, Latzin P, Ramsey KA, Stanojevic S, Aurora P, Davis SD, Gappa M, Hall GL, Horsley A, Jensen R, Lum S, Milla C, Nielsen KG, Pittman JE, Rosenfeld M, Singer F, Subbarao P, Gustafsson PM, Ratjen F; ATS Assembly on Pediatrics. Preschool Multiple-Breath Washout Testing. An Official American Thoracic Society Technical Statement. Am J Respir Crit Care Med. 2018; 197:e1-e19. doi:10.1164/rccm.201801-0074ST.

Ronan NJ, Einarsson GG, Twomey M, Mooney D, Mullane D, NiChroinin M, O'Callaghan G, Shanahan F, Murphy DM, O'Connor OJ, Shortt CA, Tunney MM, Eustace JA, Maher MM, Elborn JS, Plant BJ. CORK Study in Cystic Fibrosis: Sustained improvements in ultra-low-dose chest CT scores after CFTR modulation with ivacaftor. Chest. 2018;153:395-403. doi: 10.1016/j.chest.2017.10.005.

Rosenfeld M, Wainwright CE, Higgins M, Wang LT, McKee C, Campbell D, Tian S, Schneider J, Cunningham S, Davies JC; ARRIVAL study group. Ivacaftor treatment of cystic fibrosis in children aged 12 to <24 months and with a CFTR gating mutation (ARRIVAL): a phase 3 single-arm study. Lancet Respir Med. 2018;6:545-553. doi: 10.1016/S2213-2600(18)30202-9.

Rosenow T, Oudraad MC, Murray CP, Turkovic L, Kuo W, de Bruijne M, Ranganathan SC, Tiddens HA, Stick SM; Australian Respiratory Early Surveillance Team for Cystic Fibrosis (AREST CF). PRAGMA-CF. A quantitative structural lung disease computed tomography outcome in young children with cystic fibrosis. Am J Respir Crit Care Med. 2015;191:1158-65. doi: 10.1164/rccm.201501-0061OC.

Saunders C, Jensen R, Robinson PD, Stanojevic S, Klingel M, Short C, Davies JC, Ratjen F. Integrating the multiple breath washout test into international multicentre trials. J Cyst Fibros. 2020;19:602-607. doi: 10.1016/j.jcf.2019.11.006.

Sheikh SI, Long FR, McCoy KS, Johnson T, Ryan-Wenger NA, Hayes D Jr. Ivacaftor improves appearance of sinus disease on computerised tomography in cystic fibrosis patients with G551D mutation. Clin Otolaryngol. 2015;40:16-21. doi: 10.1111/coa.12310.

Sly PD, Brennan S, Gangell C, de Klerk N, Murray C, Mott L, Stick SM, Robinson PJ, Robertson CF, Ranganathan SC; Australian Respiratory Early Surveillance Team for Cystic Fibrosis (AREST-CF). Lung disease at diagnosis in infants with cystic fibrosis detected by newborn screening. Am J Respir Crit Care Med. 2009;180: 146-52. doi: 10.1164/rccm.200901-0069OC.

Stahl M, Joachim C, Blessing K, Hämmerling S, Sommerburg O, Latzin P, Mall MA. Multiple breath washout is feasible in the clinical setting and detects abnormal lung function in infants and young children with cystic fibrosis. Respiration. 2014;87(5):357-63. doi: 10.1159/000357075.

Stahl M, Wielpütz MO, Graeber SY, Joachim C, Sommerburg O, Kauczor HU, Puderbach M, Eichinger M, Mall MA. Comparison of lung clearance index and magnetic resonance imaging for assessment of lung disease in children with cystic fibrosis. Am J Respir Crit Care Med. 2017;195:349-359. doi: 10.1164/rccm.201604-0893OC.

Stahl M, Graeber SY, Joachim C, Barth S, Ricklefs I, Diekmann G, Kopp MV, Naehrlich L, Mall MA. Three-center feasibility of lung clearance index in infants and preschool children with cystic fibrosis and other lung diseases. J Cyst Fibros. 2018;17:249-255. doi: 10.1016/j.jcf.2017.08.001.

Stahl M, Wielpütz MO, Ricklefs I, Dopfer C, Barth S, Schlegtendal A, Graeber SY, Sommerburg O, Diekmann G, Hüsing J, Koerner-Rettberg C, Nährlich L, Dittrich AM, Kopp MV, Mall MA. Preventive inhalation of hypertonic saline in infants with cystic fibrosis (PRESIS). A randomized, double-blind, controlled study. Am J Respir Crit Care Med. 2019; 199:1238-1248. doi:10.1164/rccm.201807-1203OC.

Stahl M, Joachim C, Kirsch I, Uselmann T, Yu Y, Alfeis N, Berger C, Minso R, Rudolf I, Stolpe C, Bovermann X, Liboschik L, Steinmetz A, Tennhardt D, Dörfler F, Röhmel J, Unorji-Frank K, Rückes-Nilges C, von Stoutz B, Naehrlich L, Kopp MV, Dittrich AM, Sommerburg O, Mall MA. Multicentre feasibility of multiple-breath washout in preschool children with cystic fibrosis and other lung diseases. ERJ Open Res. 2020;6:00408-2020. doi:10.1183/23120541.00408-2020.

Stanojevic S, Davis SD, Perrem L, Shaw M, Retsch-Bogart G, Davis M, Jensen R, Clem CC, Isaac SM, Guido J, Jara S, France L, McDonald N, Solomon M, Sweezey N, Grasemann H, Waters V, Sanders DB, Ratjen FA. Determinants of lung disease progression measured by lung clearance index in children with cystic fibrosis. Eur Respir J. 2021;58:2003380. doi: 10.1183/13993003.03380-2020.

Sturgess J, Imrie J. Quantitative evaluation of the development of tracheal submucosal glands in infants with cystic fibrosis and control infants. Am J Pathol. 1982; 106:303-11.

Tabori H, Arnold C, Jaudszus A, Mentzel HJ, Renz DM, Reinsch S, Lorenz M, Michl R, Gerber A, Lehmann T, Mainz JG. Abdominal symptoms in cystic fibrosis and their relation to genotype, history, clinical and laboratory findings. PLoS One. 2017a;12:e0174463. doi: 10.1371/journal.pone.0174463

Tabori H, Jaudszus A, Arnold C, Mentzel HJ, Lorenz M, Michl RK, Lehmann T, Renz DM, Mainz JG. Relation of ultrasound findings and abdominal symptoms obtained with the CFAbd-Score in cystic fibrosis patients. Sci Rep. 2017b;7:17465. doi: 10.1038/s41598-017-17302-4.

Thomen RP, Sheshadri A, Quirk JD, Kozlowski J, Ellison HD, Szczesniak RD, Castro M, Woods JC. Regional ventilation changes in severe asthma after bronchial thermoplasty with (3)He MR imaging and CT. Radiology. 2015;274:250-9. doi: 10.1148/radiol.14140080.

Tiddens HAWM, Andrinopoulou ER, McIntosh J, Elborn JS, Kerem E, Bouma N, Bosch J, Kemner-van de Corput M. Chest computed tomography outcomes in a randomized clinical trial in cystic fibrosis: Lessons learned from the first ataluren phase 3 study. PLoS One. 2020;15:e0240898. doi: 10.1371/journal.pone.0240898.

Voskrebenzev A, Gutberlet M, Klimeš F, Kaireit TF, Schönfeld C, Rotärmel A, Wacker F, Vogel-Claussen J. Feasibility of quantitative regional ventilation and perfusion mapping with phase-resolved functional lung (PREFUL) MRI in healthy volunteers and COPD, CTEPH, and CF patients. Magn Reson Med. 2018;79: 2306-2314. doi: 10.1002/mrm.26893.

Voskrebenzev A, Vogel-Claussen J. Proton MRI of the lung: How to tame scarce protons and fast signal decay. J Magn Reson Imaging. 2021;53:1344-1357. doi: 10.1002/jmri.27122.

Wainwright CE, Vidmar S, Armstrong DS, Byrnes CA, Carlin JB, Cheney J, Cooper PJ, Grimwood K, Moodie M, Robertson CF, Tiddens HA; ACFBAL Study Investigators. Effect of bronchoalveolar lavage-directed therapy on *Pseudomonas aeruginosa* infection and structural lung injury in children with cystic fibrosis: a randomized trial. JAMA. 2011;306:163-71. doi: 10.1001/jama.2011.954.

Weatherly MR, Palmer CG, Peters ME, Green CG, Fryback D, Langhough R, Farrell PM. Wisconsin cystic fibrosis chest radiograph scoring system. Pediatrics. 1993; 91:488-95.

Wielpütz MO, Puderbach M, Kopp-Schneider A, Stahl M, Fritzsching E, Sommerburg O, Ley S, Sumkauskaite M, Biederer J, Kauczor HU, Eichinger M, Mall MA. Magnetic resonance imaging detects changes in structure and perfusion, and response to therapy in early cystic fibrosis lung disease. Am J Respir Crit Care Med. 2014;189:956-65.

Zemanick ET, Taylor-Cousar JL, Davies J, Gibson RL, Mall MA, McKone EF, McNally P, Ramsey BW, Rayment JH, Rowe SM, Tullis E, Ahluwalia N, Chu C, Ho T, Moskowitz SM, Noel S, Tian S, Waltz D, Weinstock TG, Xuan F, Wainwright CE, McColley SA. A phase 3 open-label study of Elexacaftor/Tezacaftor/Ivacaftor in children 6 through 11 years of age with cystic fibrosis and at least one F508del allele. Am J Respir Crit Care Med. 2021; 203:1522-1532. doi: 10.1164/rccm.202102-0509OC.

Zucker EJ, Barnes ZA, Lungren MP, Shpanskaya Y, Seekins JM, Halabi SS, Larson DB. Deep learning to automate Brasfield chest radiographic scoring for cystic fibrosis. J Cyst Fibros. 2020;19:131-138. doi: 10.1016/j.jcf.2019.04.016.

4. Correctors of nonsense mutations: Molecular principles, preclinical and clinical trials

Yifat S Oren, Michal Irony-Tur Sinai, Eitan Kerem, and Batsheva Kerem

4.1. Read-through of premature termination codons

About 13% of all inherited diseases as well as many cancers result from nonsense mutations leading to premature termination codons (PTCs; Linde and Kerem, 2008; Bordeira-Carriço et al., 2012). In recent years an extensive effort has been made to develop therapeutic approaches for in frame PTCs designed to promote translational read-through of the PTC and generate full length functional proteins. Compounds able to facilitate near cognate amino-acyl-tRNA incorporation (Keeling et al., 2012) can lead potentially to restoration of a functional full-length protein. If enough PTCs are converted to sense codons, sufficient full-length protein might be produced to provide a therapeutic benefit, given that the protein is functional (Oren et al., 2017). The best characterized read-through drugs are aminoglycoside antibiotics (Burke et al., 1985; Martin et al., 1989), which in addition to their antimicrobial activity by inhibition of bacterial protein synthesis (Davies et al., 1965), can also induce misreading during eukaryotic protein synthesis (Singh et al., 1979; Palmer et al., 1979). Aminoglycosides bind to the decoding site (also known as the A-site) of the 16S or 18S ribosomal RNA (rRNA) in prokaryotes and eukaryotes, respectively (Lynch et al., 2003), leading to a translation misreading (Linda and Kerem, 2008). The binding to the decoding site generates a local conformational change that mimics the change in the rRNA induced by a correct codon-anticodon pairing during translation (Vincens and Westhof, 2001). In prokaryotes this binding is efficient and therefore leads to translation inhibition. In eukaryotes the binding is less efficient, due to subtle differences in the sequence of the rRNA decoding site, and thus leads to translational read-through of PTCs by insertion of an amino acid at the stop codon (Burke and Mogg, 1985; Martin et al., 1989; van der Peer et al., 1994; Fourmy et al., 1996; Recht et al., 1996; Fan-Minogue et al., 2007). Hence, protein translation can continue to the normal end of the transcript and a full-length protein is generated with either the correct amino acid or a missense mutation (☞ Figure 4.1). Since aminoglycoside binding to the A-site is inefficient, truncated proteins are still synthesized. It is important to note that aminoglycosides are expected to have minimal or no effect on normal translation termination since the normal termination of eukaryote genes frequently consists of several stop codons and the authentic stop codons are surrounded by upstream and downstream sequences that enhance the efficiency of translation termination (Bonetti et al., 1995; Brown et al., 1990; Mc Caughan et al., 1995; Namy et al., 2001). The clinical benefit of aminoglycosides was demonstrated in cystic fibrosis (CF) patients, in which intranasal or intravenous gentamicin administration restored the CFTR-dependent Cl^- secretion and protein expression together with improved clinical end-points (Wilschanski et al., 2003; Sermet-Gaudelus et al., 2007). Unfortunately, gentamicin cannot be used as a read-through drug, due to serious renal toxicity and ototoxicity when used for prolonged periods (Oren et al., 2017).

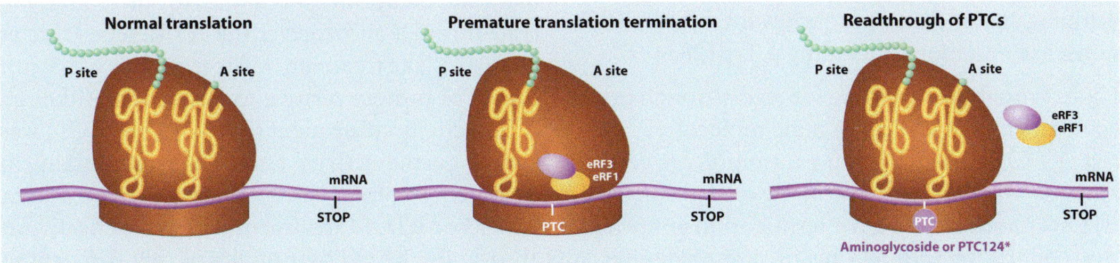

Figure 4.1: The effect of a read-through drug on protein translation (adapted from Linde and Kerem, 2008: Introducing sense into nonsense in treatments of human genetic diseases).

In an effort to enhance read-through and reduce the toxic effects of clinically used antibiotics, several derivatives of aminoglycosides have been synthesized in which the structural elements that induce toxicity were removed. These derivatives, such as NB30, NB54, NB74 and NB84, are significantly less toxic to the cells; moreover, some exhibit higher suppression efficiency than gentamicin (Brendel et al., 2011; Lee et al., 2012). NB30 promoted moderate suppression of nonsense mutations, while NB54 demonstrated a significant read-through potency in several human CF cell lines and in primary human airway cells. Moreover, NB54 restored CFTR expression and function in comparable levels as gentamicin in transgenic mice expressing a human CFTR-p.Gly542 Ter cDNA (Rowe et al., 2011). However, further *in vivo* experiments need to be carried out to analyze the nephrotoxicity and ototoxicty as well as the read-through potential of these compounds before using them for read-through therapy.

ELX-02 is a novel small molecule, non-antibiotic aminoglycoside analogue, also referred to as NB124. ELOX-02 is being developed to promote read-through of PTCs in genetic diseases (Crawford et al., 2021). ELX-02 was found to be well tolerated with pharmacokinetics properties in Phase 1 clinical trials (Leubitz et al., 2019). Phase 2 clinical trials with ELX-02 have recently initiated in CF patients carrying at least one allele of the nonsense CFTR mutation p.Gly542Ter (Kerem, 2020). The potential of ELX-02 as read-through drug was evaluated in FRT and human epithelial bronchial cells carrying the p.Gly542Ter mutation (Crawford et al., 2021) and in patient derived organoids carrying the p.Gly542Ter mutation, showing partial restoration of the CFTR function (☞ Chapter 2.4.). Currently, ELX-02 is being developed only for individuals carrying the *CFTR* p.Gly542Ter mutation, thus highlighting the importance of developing therapeutic approaches for other *CFTR* nonsense mutations, including p.Trp1282Ter.

High throughput screening for read-through molecules identified a small organic molecule, Ataluren (PTC124), which has no antibiotic properties and was hypothesized to promote read-through of PTCs without affecting the termination at normal stop codons and without causing severe side effects (Welch et al., 2007). The ability of ataluren to promote read-through *in vivo* was assessed in mouse models of DMD (Welch et al., 2007) and CF (Du et al., 2008). Both models exhibited encouraging results indicating the potential for the use of ataluren in different diseases resulting from PTC. Results from Phase 1 studies paved the way for phase 2 clinical trials (Hirawat et al., 2007). Phase 2 clinical trials for treatment of CF were performed in the US and in Israel, however statistically significant improvement in CFTR function, expressed by electrophysiological measurements, was found only in the Israeli center (Kerem et al., 2008). A subsequent study in France enrolling children carrying nonsense mutations showed results similar to the Israeli center (Sermet-Gaudelus et al., 2010). Even though, results from a phase 3 international multicenter double blind placebo controlled trial failed to achieve the primary or secondary endpoints (change in FEV1 and rate of exacerbations) and the clinical development of ataluren was discontinued.

4.2. Novel drug developments

In an attempt to discover drugs with increased read-through activity and reduced toxicity relative to aminoglycosides, various molecules have been identified, among them negamycin, a dipeptide antibiotic that was tested in *mdx* mice and showed a less toxic effect than gentamicin *in vivo*. Acetylamino benzoic acid was examined in cell culture and *mdx* mice. This compound enables read-through of nonsense mutations in lower concentrations as compared to G418. Clitocin is a nucleoside analog whose read-through potency was assessed in several human cancer cell lines with PTCs in the *P53* gene and in a xenograft model. Clitocin treatment was more effective than G418 in cell lines and inhibited cancer growth *in vivo*. RTC13 and RTC14 are two low molecular-weight read-through compounds that were tested in lymphoblastoid and fibroblast cell lines for their ability to read-through and correct the *ATM* gene (Xue et al., 2014). The treatment led to synthesis of $\leq$5% of the ATM protein relative to WT levels. Although ATM activity subsequent to RTC13 or RTC14 was similar to the activity after G418 or gentamicin treatment, colony survival assay showed that RTC13 or RTC14 treatment was more effective at abrogating the radiosensitivity of cells deficient in ATM activity than G418, and in a lower concentration.

Screening of a library of 1,600 clinically approved compounds led to the identification of Escin, an herbal agent with anti-inflammatory, anti-edematous and vasoprotective properties. Escin elicited increased levels of read-through, demonstrated by enhanced CFTR expression and function in CF primary human bronchial epithelial (HBE) cells carrying the p.Gly542Ter mutation (Mutyam et al., 2016).

Recently, a screen of thousands of compounds identified SRI-37240 and its more potent derivative SRI-41315. These small molecules were shown to induce a prolonged pause at stop codons by reducing the level of the termination factor eRF1, enabling read-through activity. Furthermore, SRI-41315 also potentiated aminoglycoside-mediated read-through, leading to synergistic increases in CFTR activity in immortalized and primary HBE cells. However, these molecules had undesirable effects on sodium transport by ENaC that limit their immediate development for the treatment of CF (Sharma et al., 2021).

Modulating the translation termination pathway by reducing eRF1 abundance as a potential therapeutic approach for PTC suppression was demonstrated also by antisense oligonucleotide (ASO)-mediated knockdown. ASO-mediated partial reduction of either eRF1 or eRF3a in the mouse liver in Haemophilia mice expressing a mutant allele of human coagulation factor IX carrying the p.Arg 338Ter mutation. Both ASOs worked in synergy with geneticin, a small molecule read-through drug, demonstrating significantly increased production of functional full length hFIX protein to levels that would rescue disease phenotypes in these mice (Huang et al., 2019).

Various macrolides exhibit read-through activity and were shown to reduce the oncogenic phenotype of colorectal cancer cells and a xenograft model harboring PTC in the *APC* gene(Lee et al., 2012). The read-through efficacy of the macrolide Azithromycin was demonstrated in the severe mouse model of spinal muscular atrophy (SMA). A low dose of Azithromycin was able to increase SMN protein and impact disease severity (Osman et al., 2017). Although more extensive studies should be performed to elucidate the mode of activity of these compounds, their potency and side effects, the preliminary results show the potential of using these compounds for read-through therapies.

Another novel approach to read-through of PTC is by suppressor tRNA. Suppressor-tRNA is a mutant tRNA with an anticodon sequence that is complementary to a stop codon. Incorporation of an amino acid at the stop codon by this suppressor-tRNA enables read-through of the PTC and synthesis of the full-length protein. Suppressor-tRNA was shown to be effective in read-through of PTC *in vitro* for xeroderma pigmentosum, thalassemia and DMD (Bordeira-Carriço et al., 2012). Additionally, suppressor-tRNA restored the COL6A protein expression in Ullrich patients' fibroblasts, which is indicative of the therapeutic potential of suppressor tRNA (Sako et al., 2006). However, it is important to note that the *in vivo* delivery of the tRNA-suppressor vector may be difficult.

A novel strategy for the CFTR p.Trp1282Ter mutation is the use of ASO to skip over the exon harboring the severe mutation in the CFTR transcript to produce functional proteins. Since this exon is in frame, it could be removed without causing a frameshift. The results show that the selected lead ASOs significantly decreased the level of CFTR transcripts with exon 23 and thereby bypassed the p.Trp1282Ter mutation that subjects the CFTR transcripts to Nonsense Mediated mRNA Decay (NMD) and the truncated proteins to degradation (Linde et al., 2007; Mutyam et al., 2017). As a result of the ASO treatment, a significant level of CFTR protein was produced and maturated and together with elexacaftor/tezacaftor/ivacaftor (☞ Chapter 5.) a significant activation of the CFTR channel was demonstrated.

4.3. The role of CFTR modulators as a therapeutic approach for *CFTR* nonsense mutations

Since read-through promotes incorporation of near cognate amino acid, the resulted proteins can be misfolded or present a defective activity. Indeed, pairing read-through agents with clinically approved Vertex CFTR modulators enhanced their function (Mutyam et al., 2016; Haggie et al., 2017; Xue et al., 2017). Ivacaftor (☞ Chapter 5.) alone had a modest but detectable clinical benefit in a CF patient homozygous for p.Trp1282Ter mutation (Mutyam et al., 2017). As CFTR read-through products exhibit a mix of missense mutations caused by insertion of near-cognate amino acids, CFTR modulators that maximally correct or potentiate nonsense mutations after PTC suppression are needed in order to achieve clinically beneficial response. Recently, a series of novel CFTR modulators were identified, among them C1 and C2, novel corrector molecules that have complementary mode of action and are more efficient than lumacaftor in rescuing the F508del allele (de Wilde et al., 2019). GLPG1837 is a novel potentiator that went through a clinical trial in patients with p.Gly551Asp or p.Ser1251Asn *CFTR* gating mutations. This compound exerting activity both on its own and in combination with correctors (Davies et al., 2019). The combination of C1, C2 and GLPG1837 alone and in combination with G418 as translational read-through improved CFTR function in cell lines and patient derived primary HBE cells and organoids, all carrying nonsense mutations in the *CFTR* gene (Mutyam et al., 2021). These results indicate a role for CFTR modulation as a therapeutic approach for CF patients carrying nonsense mutations, although efficacy may ultimately be limited by the low levels of transcripts observed in patients resulting from NMD (Linde et al., 2007).

4.4. Variability in the response to read-through treatment

Read-through studies using aminoglycosides or ataluren have revealed variable responses to treatment among CF patients (Wilschanski et al., 2000; 2003; Kerem et al., 2008; Clancy et al., 2007). A variable response was also observed among DMD patients carrying a PTC in the *dystrophin* gene and in a mouse model of DMD (Barton-Davis et al., 1999; Dunant et al., 2003; Wagner et al., 2001; Politano et al., 2003). Variability in response to read-through treatment may result from:

- **I.** Differences in the identity of the PTC and its sequence context. Using reporter constructs it was shown that the levels of read-through are correlated with established translation termination efficiencies. The highest read-through efficiency is the UGA stop codon, followed by UAG and to a lesser extent UAA (Manuvakhova et al., 2000; Howard et al., 2000). These studies also showed that the sequences upstream and downstream to the stop codon play an important role in determining its susceptibility to read-through (Bidou et al., 2004).
- **II.** Differences in the chemical composition of the aminoglycoside. Comparison of read-through efficiency induced by various aminoglycosides such as gentamicin, amikacin, tobramycin, paromomycin and neomycin in human cells expressing a reporter gene with a PTC showed a higher read-through efficiency in cells treated with gentamicin and amikacin than in cells treated with the other aminoglycosides (Diop et al., 2007; Howard et al., 2004; Noensie and Dietz, 2001).
- **III.** Variability in aminoglycoside metabolism between individuals, different durations of the read-through treatment or the method of application could also account for the variable response found in different studies.

However, none of these factors can explain the differences in the response to read-through treatment in patients who participated in the same clinical study, and who carry the same PTC. Since PTC-bearing transcripts are the template for read-through, cellular processes regulating the levels of these transcripts may have a major effect on the response to the treatment. The first step towards revealing the molecular basis for the variable response to read-through treatments involved analyzing the CFTR transcripts levels in patients carrying the same PTC (p.Trp1282Ter). Substantial variability among patients in the transcript level was found, which was correlated with their response. Specifically, a response was found only in patients with relatively high levels of CFTR transcripts, whereas no response was found in patients with markedly reduced levels (Linde et al., 2007). This result suggests that the transcript level is a limiting factor of the response. Different cellular mechanisms can regulate the levels of transcripts carrying PTC, including the NMD and the Unfolded Protein Response (UPR).

4.5. NMD as a regulator of the response to read-through treatment

Transcripts carrying PTCs are subjected to degradation by the NMD mechanism. Since these transcripts are the template for read-through treatment, it was suggested that the NMD regulates the read-through response. Inhibition of NMD by siRNA directed against NMD key factors (UPF1 or UPF2) in cell lines carrying PTC in the CFTR gene led to an increased level of CFTR nonsense transcripts. Importantly, CFTR chloride channel activity improved in gentamicin-treated cells in which UPF1 or UPF2 was downregulated compared to cells treated with gentamicin alone (Linde et al., 2007). These results support the general view that NMD affects the level of nonsense transcripts and regulates the response to gentamicin. Variability in NMD efficiency has been found in cell lines, tissues and among individuals, indicating that the efficiency of NMD is an inherent character of cells (Holbrook et al., 2004; Linde et al., 2007). Various mechanisms were found to control NMD efficiency, among them the exon sequence downstream of the PTC, the PTC-to-intron distance, and the number of introns both upstream and downstream of the PTC (Hoek et al., 2019). It was also described that a subpopulation of mRNA molecules can escape NMD, further affecting NMD efficiency. This variability may affect the level of PTC-bearing transcripts available for read-through treatment, leading to variable response to read-through treatment among patients. Hence the NMD mechanism plays an important role in modulating the response to read-through treatments (Linde and Kerem, 2008; Kuzmiak and Maquat, 2006; Schweingruber et al., 2013). Understanding the molecular mechanism governing NMD and the physiological and environmental conditions that regulate its efficiency is important for developing therapeutic approaches aimed specifically at manipulating NMD efficiency (Schweingruber et al., 2013). Any process that inhibits NMD and enables nonsense-containing transcripts to be resistant to NMD degradation will result in higher levels of these transcripts, which can then be the template for read-through treatment. In an attempt to identify NMD inhibitors, the small molecule amlexanox was identified (Gonzalez-Hilarion et al., 2012). Interestingly, amlexanox was shown to display a dual activity of both readthrouth and NMD inhibition, leading to the synthesis of full-length proteins in an efficient manner. However, in a recently published work, Amlexanox did not cause sufficient readthrough to restore functional levels of CFTR in primary cells from a mouse model carrying a p.Gly542Ter nonsense mutation in the *CFTR* gene (McHugh et al., 2020). In a more recent study, NMD inhibition by down regulating the expression of the NMD factor SMG1, led to upregulation of the Trp1282Ter mRNA and surface-localized protein expression of the truncated Trp1282Ter gene product in a HEK293 minigene model. Moreover, SMG1 inhibition in a human bronchial epithelial cell line homozygous for the p.Trp1282Ter mutation, increased Trp1282Ter mRNA, protein and function (Keenan et al., 2019). Using intestinal organoids (☞ Chapter 2.4.), a partial rescue of the Trp1282 Ter-CFTR function was achieved with SMG1 inhibition combined with ELX-02 readthrough and the CFTR-modulators elexacaftor/tezacaftor/ivacaftor. A variation in the level of CFTR functional rescue was observed between different p.Trp1282Ter homozygous organoids, still all cultures reached swelling levels comparable to the limited rescue of p.Phe508del/p.Phe508del organoids with lumacaftor/ivacaftor, highlighting the need for a combination of pharmacotherapies to rescue PTC (de Poel et al., 2021).

As NMD regulates the expression of many genes (Mendell et al., 2004), a transcript specific stabilization is needed for the development of a therapeutic approach. Such approach was adapted for the CFTR Trp1282Ter transcripts by using a cocktail of three ASOs designed to prevent binding of exon junction complexes (EJC) downstream of the PTC. These ASOs specifically increases the expression of CFTR Trp1282Ter mRNA leading to increased levels of truncated CFTR protein and CFTR function in human bronchial epithelial cell line (Kim et al., 2021).

4.6. UPR as a regulator of the response to read-through treatment

Increasing evidence shows that cellular stresses lead to reduced NMD efficiency (Gardner and Corn, 2008; Gardner, 2010; Volkmann et al., 2011). One example is ER stress activating the UPR which alters the transcriptional and translational cellular programs, including attenuation of translation (Harding et al., 1999; Wek et al., 2006). Since the NMD is a translation-dependent mechanism (Nicholson et al., 2010), it was indeed shown that UPR activation inhibits the NMD mechanism

(Wang et al., 2011; Oren et al., 2014). Specifically, UPR activation led to a significant increase in the level of transcripts carrying disease-causing PTCs in cell lines derived from patients carrying PTCs in the *CFTR*, XRCC4-like factor (*XLF*), and *LPIN1* genes. Furthermore, UPR activation enabled the correction of the CFTR and XLF function following read-through treatment (Oren et al., 2014). Interestingly, quantitative proteomic analyses showed substantial differences in UPR activation among patients carrying the same PTCs in the *CFTR* gene, which is correlated with their response to the read-through treatment (Oren et al., 2014). Higher levels of known ER resident proteins that are activated by the UPR were found in the cells derived from the responsive patients. The proteomic results raise the possibility that UPR plays a role in the regulation of read-through treatment for patients carrying disease-causing PTCs. Thus, the variability in response to the read-through treatment could have resulted from a difference in activation of UPR, leading to variable NMD efficiency. Consequently, higher UPR activation could account for the differences in PTC-carrying transcript levels which led to the differential response to read-through treatments. Strikingly, NMD inhibition was found to activate the UPR due to accumulation of truncated proteins in the ER. In fact, a significant inverse correlation between the UPR and NMD was found among CF patients, suggesting a feedback loop between these homeostatic pathways. This feedback loop augments both UPR activation and NMD inhibition and therefore enhances the response to read-through treatment (Oren et al., 2014).

The variability in the response to read-through treatments found in pre-clinical and clinical studies suggests that combinational therapy using a cocktail of drugs that enable modulation of various mechanisms together may be required to enhance sufficient production of full-length functional protein. For example, this could involve modulating gene expression (Rowe et al., 2007), NMD efficiency (Gonzalez-Hilarion et al., 2012; Durand et al., 2007), or activating the UPR (Oren et al., 2014) together with read-through treatment. Revealing tissue specific UPR and NMD inducers is expected to provide a new therapeutic approach to improve patients' response to read-through treatment. Additionally, a combination of different types of read-through compounds to reduce toxicity while improving read-through efficiency might be beneficial as well (Lee and Dougherty, 2012). These could potentially lead to customized therapy for individual patients.

The novel bidirectional crosstalk between NMD and the UPR was further established in various cellular models. Karam et al. reported that NMD determines the threshold of UPR activation, shaping its timely termination to control cell fate under ER stress (Karam et al., 2015). The authors examined in HeLa cells with disrupted NMD pathway the mRNA levels of a variety of UPR components, and found that the highly conserved UPR sensor, IRE1α, was one of the most induced genes at the mRNA and protein levels. The identification of mRNAs encoding UPR components that are targeted for decay by NMD validates that NMD perturbation triggers ER stress and demonstrates the crucial role of NMD in regulating the UPR. The ability of NMD to both regulate and shape ER-stress and non-ER stress responses was further reviewed by Goetz and Wilkinson (2017) and raises the possibility that NMD modulatory therapy could be clinically beneficial in some disease settings, including cancer and neurodegeneration.

Using a quantitative assay for monitoring changes in individual NMD-sensitive isoforms, Li et al. (2017) revealed a strong correlation between NMD inhibition, ER stress and polysome disassembly upon thapsigargin treatment in a temporal and dose-dependent manner. Their results demonstrated the necessity of PERK activation as well as the strong correlation between polysome disassembly and NMD inhibition and revealed that different NMD targets have varying sensitivity to NMD inactivation (Li et al., 2017).

Recently, a localized NMD pathway dedicated to ER-translated mRNAs was identified (Longman et al., 2020). The proposed model includes NBAS (neuroblastoma amplified sequence)-mediated UPF1 recruitment to the ER membrane and activation of an ER-dedicated NMD pathway, ensuring quality control of ER-translated mRNA. Altogether, these findings highlight the dynamic crosstalk between mRNA metabolism and the protein homeostasis network.

In summary, revealing the molecular basis modulating the response to read-through treatment, together with improvement in drug efficiency may pave the way to the development of read-through 'tailor made' therapies based on the sequence profile of each individual for many human diseases caused by PTCs.

Besides these mutation-type specific options, novel strategies aim to correct not one but many mutations at the same time by a mutation-agnostic approach: the targeted integration of a super-exon spanning exons 2-28 within intron 1 of the endogenous *CFTR* locus (Mention et al., 2019). In contrast to the common approach for genomic restoration of CFTR that the sequence is integrated elsewhere in the genome (Guan et al., 2019), the regulation of protein expression should remain unaltered. The ultimate goal would be to target the integration of the super-exon into the *CFTR* locus of long-lived basal stem cells of the CF airway (Carraro et al., 2021; Ensinck et al., 2021; King et al., 2020).

4.7. References

Barton-Davis ER, Cordier L, Shoturma DI, Leland SE, Sweeney HL. Aminoglycoside antibiotics restore dystrophin function to skeletal muscles of mdx mice. J Clin Invest. 1999;104:375-81. doi: 10.1172/JCI7866.

Bidou L, Hatin I, Perez N, Allamand V, Panthier JJ, Rousset JP. Premature stop codons involved in muscular dystrophies show a broad spectrum of readthrough efficiencies in response to gentamicin treatment. Gene Ther. 2004;11:619-27. doi: 10.1038/sj.gt.3302211.

Bonetti B, Fu L, Moon J, Bedwell DM. The efficiency of translation termination is determined by a synergistic interplay between upstream and downstream sequences in *Saccharomyces cerevisiae.* J Mol Biol. 1995;251:334-45. doi: 10.1006/jmbi.1995.0438.

Bordeira-Carriço R, Pêgo AP, Santos M, Oliveira C. Cancer syndromes and therapy by stop-codon readthrough. Trends Mol Med 2012;18:667-78. doi://doi.org/10.1016/j.molmed.2012.09.004.

Brendel C, Belakhov V, Werner H, Wegener E, Gärtner J, Nudelman I, Baasov T, Huppke P. Readthrough of nonsense mutations in Rett syndrome: evaluation of novel aminoglycosides and generation of a new mouse model. J Mol Med (Berl). 2011;89:389-98. doi: 10.1007/s00109-010-0704-4.

Brown CM, Stockwell PA, Trotman CN, Tate WP. Sequence analysis suggests that tetra-nucleotides signal the termination of protein synthesis in eukaryotes. Nucleic Acids Res. 1990;18:6339-45. doi: 10.1093/nar/18.21.6339.

Burke JF, Mogg AE. Suppression of a nonsense mutation in mammalian cells in vivo by the aminoglycoside antibiotics G-418 and paromomycin. Nucleic Acids Res 1985; 13:6265–72. doi: 10.1093/nar/13.17.6265.

Carraro G, Langerman J, Sabri S, Lorenzana Z, Purkayastha A, Zhang G, Konda B, Aros CJ, Calvert BA, Szymaniak A, Wilson E, Mulligan M, Bhatt P, Lu J, Vijayaraj P, Yao C, Shia DW, Lund AJ, Israely E, Rickabaugh TM, Ernst J, Mense M, Randell SH, Vladar EK, Ryan AL, Plath K, Mahoney JE, Stripp BR, Gomperts BN. Transcriptional analysis of cystic fibrosis airways at single-cell resolution reveals altered epithelial cell states and composition. Nat Med. 2021;27:806-814. doi: 10.1038/s41591-021-01332-7.

Carreras-Sureda A, Hetz C. RNA metabolism: putting the brake on the UPR. EMBO Rep. 2015;16:545-6. doi: 10.15252/embr.201540227.

Clancy JP, Rowe SM, Bebok Z, Aitken ML, Gibson R, Zeitlin P, Berclaz P, Moss R, Knowles MR, Oster RA, Mayer-Hamblett N, Ramsey B. No detectable improvements in cystic fibrosis transmembrane conductance regulator by nasal aminoglycosides in patients with cystic fibrosis with stop mutations. Am J Respir Cell Mol Biol. 2007; 37:57-66. doi: 10.1165/rcmb.2006-0173OC.

Crawford DK, Mullenders J, Pott J, Boj SF, Landskroner-Eiger S, Goddeeris MM. Targeting G542X CFTR nonsense alleles with ELX-02 restores CFTR function in human-derived intestinal organoids. J Cyst Fibros. 2021;20: 436-442. doi: 10.1016/j.jcf.2021.01.009.

Davies J, Gorini L, Davis BD. Misreading of RNA codewords induced by aminoglycoside antibiotics. Mol Pharmacol. 1965;1:93-106

Davies JC, Van de Steen O, van Koningsbruggen-Rietschel S, Drevinek P, Derichs N, McKone EF, Kanters D, Allamassey L, Namour F, de Kock H, Conrath K. GLPG1837, a CFTR potentiator, in p.Gly551Asp (G551D)-CF patients: An open-label, single-arm, phase 2a study (SAPHIRA1). J Cyst Fibros. 2019;18:693-699. doi: 10.1016/j.jcf.2019.05.006.

de Poel E, Spelier S, Suen SWF, Kruisselbrink E, Graeber SY, Mall MA, Weersink EJM, van der Eerden MM, Koppelman GH, van der Ent CK, Beekman JM. Functional restoration of CFTR nonsense mutations in intestinal organoids. J Cyst Fibros. 2021; 16:S1569-1993(21) 01425-9. doi: 10.1016/j.jcf.2021.09.020.

de Wilde G, Gees M, Musch S, Verdonck K, Jans M, Wesse AS, Singh AK, Hwang TC, Christophe T, Pizzonero M, Van der Plas S, Desroy N, Cowart M, Stouten P, Nelles L, Conrath K. Identification of GLPG/ABBV-2737, a novel class of corrector, which exerts functional synergy with other CFTR modulators. Front Pharmacol. 2019;10:514. doi: 10.3389/fphar.2019.00514.

Diop D, Chauvin C, Jean-Jean O. Aminoglycosides and other factors promoting stop codon readthrough in human cells. C R Biol. 2007;330:71-9. doi: 10.1016/j.crvi.2006.09.001.

Du M, Liu X, Welch EM, Hirawat S, Peltz SW, Bedwell DM. PTC124 is an orally bioavailable compound that promotes suppression of the human CFTR-G542X nonsense allele in a CF mouse model. Proc Natl Acad Sci U S A. 2008;105:2064-9. doi: 10.1073/pnas.0711795105.

Dunant P, Walter MC, Karpati G, Lochmüller H. Gentamicin fails to increase dystrophin expression in dystrophin-deficient muscle. Muscle Nerve. 2003;27:624-7. doi: 10.1002/mus.10341.

Durand S, Cougot N, Mahuteau-Betzer F, Nguyen CH, Grierson DS, Bertrand E, Tazi J, Lejeune F. Inhibition of nonsense-mediated mRNA decay (NMD) by a new chemical molecule reveals the dynamic of NMD factors in P-bodies. J Cell Biol. 2007; 178:1145-60. doi: 10.1083/jcb.200611086.

Ensinck M, Mottais A, Detry C, Leal T, Carlon MS. On the corner of models and cure: Gene editing in cystic fibrosis. Front Pharmacol. 2021;12:662110. doi: 10.3389/fphar.2021.662110.

Fan-Minogue H, Bedwell DM. Eukaryotic ribosomal RNA determinants of aminoglycoside resistance and their role in translational fidelity. RNA. 2008; 14:148-57. doi: 10.1261/rna.805208.

Fourmy D, Recht MI, Blanchard SC, Puglisi JD. Structure of the A site of *Escherichia coli* 16S ribosomal RNA complexed with an aminoglycoside antibiotic. Science. 1996; 274:1367-71. doi: 10.1126/science.274.5291.1367.

Gardner LB. Nonsense-mediated RNA decay regulation by cellular stress: implications for tumorigenesis. Mol Cancer Res. 2010;8:295-308. doi: 10.1158/1541-7786.MCR-09-0502.

Gardner LB, Corn PG. Hypoxic regulation of mRNA expression. Cell Cycle. 2008; 7:1916-24. doi: 10.4161/cc.7.13.6203.

Goetz AE, Wilkinson M. Stress and the nonsense-mediated RNA decay pathway. Cell Mol Life Sci. 2017; 74:3509-3531. doi: 10.1007/s00018-017-2537-6.

Gonzalez-Hilarion S, Beghyn T, Jia J, Debreuck N, Berte G, Mamchaoui K, Mouly V, Gruenert DC, Déprez B, Lejeune F. Rescue of nonsense mutations by amlexanox in human cells. Orphanet J Rare Dis. 2012;7:58. doi: 10.1186/1750-1172-7-58.

Guan S, Munder A, Hedtfeld S, Braubach P, Glage S, Zhang L, Lienenklaus S, Schultze A, Hasenpusch G, Garrels W, Stanke F, Miskey C, Johler SM, Kumar Y, Tümmler B, Rudolph C, Ivics Z, Rosenecker J. Self-assembled peptide-poloxamine nanoparticles enable in vitro and in vivo genome restoration for cystic fibrosis. Nat Nanotechnol. 2019;14:287-297. doi: 10.1038/s41565-018-0358-x.

Haggie PM, Phuan PW, Tan JA, Xu H, Avramescu RG, Perdomo D, Zlock L, Nielson DW, Finkbeiner WE, Lukacs GL, Verkman AS. Correctors and potentiators rescue function of the truncated W1282X-Cystic Fibrosis Transmembrane Regulator (CFTR) translation product. J Biol Chem. 2017;292:771-785. doi: 10.1074/jbc.M116.764720.

Harding HP, Zhang Y, Ron D. Protein translation and folding are coupled by an endoplasmic-reticulum-resident kinase. Nature. 1999;397:271-4. doi: 10.1038/16729.

Hirawat S, Welch EM, Elfring GL, Northcutt VJ, Paushkin S, Hwang S, Leonard EM, Almstead NG, Ju W, Peltz SW, Miller LL. Safety, tolerability, and pharmacokinetics of PTC124, a nonaminoglycoside nonsense mutation suppressor, following single- and multiple-dose administration to healthy male and female adult volunteers. J Clin Pharmacol. 2007;47:430-44. doi: 10.1177/0091270006297140.

Holbrook JA, Neu-Yilik G, Hentze MW, Kulozik AE. Nonsense-mediated decay approaches the clinic. Nat Genet. 2004;36:801-8. doi: 10.1038/ng1403.

Hoek TA, Khuperkar D, Lindeboom RGH, Sonneveld S, Verhagen BMP, Boersma S, Vermeulen M, Tanenbaum ME. Single-molecule imaging uncovers rules governing nonsense-mediated mRNA decay. Mol Cell. 2019;75:324-339.e11. doi: 10.1016/j.molcel.2019.05.008.

Howard MT, Shirts BH, Petros LM, Flanigan KM, Gesteland RF, Atkins JF. Sequence specificity of aminoglycoside-induced stop condon readthrough: potential implications for treatment of Duchenne muscular dystrophy. Ann Neurol. 2000;48:164-9.

Howard MT, Anderson CB, Fass U, Khatri S, Gesteland RF, Atkins JF, Flanigan KM. Readthrough of dystrophin stop codon mutations induced by aminoglycosides. Ann Neurol. 2004;55:422-6. doi: 10.1002/ana.20052.

Huang L, Aghajan M, Quesenberry T, Low A, Murray SF, Monia BP, Guo S. Targeting translation termination machinery with antisense oligonucleotides for diseases caused by nonsense mutations. Nucleic Acid Ther. 2019; 29:175-186. doi: 10.1089/nat.2019.0779.

Karam R, Lou CH, Kroeger H, Huang L, Lin JH, Wilkinson MF. The unfolded protein response is shaped by the NMD pathway. EMBO Rep. 2015;16:599-609. doi: 10.15252/embr.201439696.

Keeling KM, Wang D, Conard SE, Bedwell DM. Suppression of premature termination codons as a therapeutic approach. Crit Rev Biochem Mol Biol 2012;47:444–63. https://doi.org/10.3109/10409238.2012.694846.

Keenan MM, Huang L, Jordan NJ, Wong E, Cheng Y, Valley HC, Mahiou J, Liang F, Bihler H, Mense M, Guo S, Monia BP. Nonsense-mediated RNA decay pathway inhibition restores expression and function of W1282X CFTR. Am J Respir Cell Mol Biol. 2019;61:290-300. doi: 10.1165/rcmb.2018-0316OC.

Kerem E. ELX-02: an investigational read-through agent for the treatment of nonsense mutation-related genetic disease. Expert Opin Investig Drugs. 2020 ; 29:1347-1354. doi: 10.1080/13543784.2020.1828862.

Kerem E, Hirawat S, Armoni S, Yaakov Y, Shoseyov D, Cohen M, Nissim-Rafinia M, Blau H, Rivlin J, Aviram M, Elfring GL, Northcutt VJ, Miller LL, Kerem B, Wilschanski M. Effectiveness of PTC124 treatment of cystic fibrosis caused by nonsense mutations: a prospective phase II trial. Lancet. 2008;372:719-27. doi: 10.1016/S0140-6736(08)61168-X.

Kim YJ, Nomakuchi T, Papaleonidopoulou ARK. Gene-specific nonsense-mediated mRNA decay targeting for cystic fibrosis therapy. BioRxiv 2021. https://doi.org/10.1101/2021.07.13. 452144.

King NE, Suzuki S, Barillà C, Hawkins FJ, Randell SH, Reynolds SD, Stripp BR, Davis BR. Correction of airway stem cells: Genome editing approaches for the treatment of cystic fibrosis. Hum Gene Ther. 2020;31:956-972. doi: 10.1089/hum.2020.160

Kuzmiak HA, Maquat LE. Applying nonsense-mediated mRNA decay research to the clinic: progress and challenges. Trends Mol Med. 2006;12:306-16. doi: 10.1016/j.molmed.2006.05.005.

Lee HL, Dougherty JP. Pharmaceutical therapies to recode nonsense mutations in inherited diseases. Pharmacol Ther. 2012;136:227-66. doi: 10.1016/j.pharmthera.2012.07.007.

Leubitz A, Frydman-Marom A, Sharpe N, van Duzer J, Campbell KCM, Vanhoutte F. Safety, tolerability, and pharmacokinetics of single ascending doses of ELX-02, a potential treatment for genetic disorders caused by nonsense mutations, in healthy volunteers. Clin Pharmacol Drug Dev. 2019;8:984-994. doi: 10.1002/cpdd.647.

Li Z, Vuong JK, Zhang M, Stork C, Zheng S. Inhibition of nonsense-mediated RNA decay by ER stress. RNA. 2017; 23:378-394. doi: 10.1261/rna.058040.116.

Linde L, Kerem B. Introducing sense into nonsense in treatments of human genetic diseases. Trends Genet 2008;24:552-63. doi: 10.1016/j.tig.2008.08.010.

Linde L, Boelz S, Nissim-Rafinia M, Oren YS, Wilschanski M, Yaacov Y, Virgilis D, Neu-Yilik G, Kulozik AE, Kerem E, Kerem B. Nonsense-mediated mRNA decay affects nonsense transcript levels and governs response of cystic fibrosis patients to gentamicin. J Clin Invest. 2007;117:683-92. doi: 10.1172/JCI28523.

Linde L, Boelz S, Neu-Yilik G, Kulozik AE, Kerem B. The efficiency of nonsense-mediated mRNA decay is an inherent character and varies among different cells. Eur J Hum Genet. 2007;15:1156-62. doi: 10.1038/sj.ejhg.5201889.

Longman D, Jackson-Jones KA, Maslon MM, Murphy LC, Young RS, Stoddart JJ, Hug N, Taylor MS, Papadopoulos DK, Cáceres JF. Identification of a localized nonsense-mediated decay pathway at the endoplasmic reticulum. Genes Dev. 2020; 34:1075-1088. doi: 10.1101/gad.338061.120.

Lynch SR, Gonzalez RL, Puglisi JD. Comparison of X-ray crystal structure of the 30S subunit-antibiotic complex with NMR structure of decoding site oligonucleotide-paromomycin complex. Structure. 2003;11:43-53. doi: 10.1016/s0969-2126(02)00934-6.

Manuvakhova M, Keeling K, Bedwell DM. Aminoglycoside antibiotics mediate context-dependent suppression of termination codons in a mammalian translation system. RNA. 2000;6:1044-55. doi: 10.1017/s1355838200000716.

Martin R, Mogg AE, Heywood LA, Nitschke L, Burke JF. Aminoglycoside suppression at UAG, UAA and UGA codons in *Escherichia coli* and human tissue culture cells. Mol Gen Genet 1989;217:411–8. doi: 10.1007/BF02464911

McCaughan KK, Brown CM, Dalphin ME, Berry MJ, Tate WP. Translational termination efficiency in mammals is influenced by the base following the stop codon. Proc Natl Acad Sci U S A. 1995;92:5431-5. doi: 10.1073/pnas.92.12.5431.

McHugh DR, Cotton CU, Hodges CA. Synergy between readthrough and nonsense mediated decay inhibition in a murine model of cystic fibrosis nonsense mutations. Int J Mol Sci. 2020;22:344. doi: 10.3390/ijms22010344.

Mendell JT, Sharifi NA, Meyers JL, Martinez-Murillo F, Dietz HC. Nonsense surveillance regulates expression of diverse classes of mammalian transcripts and mutes genomic noise. Nat Genet. 2004;36:1073-8. doi: 10.1038/ng1429.

Mention K, Santos L, Harrison PT. Gene and base editing as a therapeutic option for cystic fibrosis - Learning from other diseases. Genes (Basel). 2019;10:387. doi: 10.3390/genes10050387.

Mutyam V, Libby EF, Peng N, Hadjiliadis D, Bonk M, Solomon GM, Rowe SM. Therapeutic benefit observed with the CFTR potentiator, ivacaftor, in a CF patient homozygous for the W1282X CFTR nonsense mutation. J Cyst Fibros. 2017; 16:24-29. doi: 10.1016/j.jcf.2016.09.005.

Mutyam V, Du M, Xue X, Keeling KM, White EL, Bostwick JR, Rasmussen L, Liu B, Mazur M, Hong JS, Falk Libby E, Liang F, Shang H, Mense M, Suto MJ,

Bedwell DM, Rowe SM. Discovery of clinically approved agents that promote suppression of Cystic Fibrosis Transmembrane Conductance Regulator nonsense mutations. Am J Respir Crit Care Med. 2016;194:1092-1103. doi: 10.1164/rccm.201601-0154OC.

Mutyam V, Sharma J, Li Y, Peng N, Chen J, Tang LP, Falk Libby E, Singh AK, Conrath K, Rowe SM. Novel correctors and potentiators enhance translational readthrough in CFTR nonsense mutations. Am J Respir Cell Mol Biol. 2021;64:604-616. doi: 10.1165/rcmb.2019-0291OC.

Namy O, Hatin I, Rousset JP. Impact of the six nucleotides downstream of the stop codon on translation termination. EMBO Rep. 2001;2:787-93. doi: 10.1093/embo-reports/kve176.

Nicholson P, Yepiskoposyan H, Metze S, Zamudio Orozco R, Kleinschmidt N, Mühlemann O. Nonsense-mediated mRNA decay in human cells: mechanistic insights, functions beyond quality control and the double-life of NMD factors. Cell Mol Life Sci. 2010;67:677-700. doi: 10.1007/s00018-009-0177-1.

Noensie EN, Dietz HC. A strategy for disease gene identification through nonsense-mediated mRNA decay inhibition. Nat Biotechnol. 2001;19:434-9. doi: 10.1038/88099.

Oren YS, McClure ML, Rowe SM, Sorscher EJ, Bester AC, Manor M, Kerem E, Rivlin J, Zahdeh F, Mann M, Geiger T, Kerem B. The unfolded protein response affects readthrough of premature termination codons. EMBO Mol Med. 2014;6:685-701. doi: 10.1002/emmm.201303347.

Oren YS, Pranke IM, Kerem B, Sermet-Gaudelus I. The suppression of premature termination codons and the repair of splicing mutations in CFTR. Curr Opin Pharmacol 2017;34:125-31. https://doi.org/10.1016/j.coph.2017.09.017.

Osman EY, Washington CW, Simon ME, Megiddo D, Greif H, Lorson CL. Analysis of azithromycin monohydrate as a single or a combinatorial therapy in a mouse model of severe spinal muscular atrophy. J Neuromuscul Dis. 2017;4:237-249. doi: 10.3233/JND-170230.

Palmer E, Wilhelm JM, Sherman F. Phenotypic suppression of nonsense mutants in yeast by aminoglycoside antibiotics. Nature. 1979;277:148-50. doi: 10.1038/277148a0.

Politano L, Nigro G, Nigro V, Piluso G, Papparella S, Paciello O, Comi LI. Gentamicin administration in Duchenne patients with premature stop codon. Preliminary results. Acta Myol. 2003;22:15-21.

Recht MI, Fourmy D, Blanchard SC, Dahlquist KD, Puglisi JD. RNA sequence determinants for aminoglycoside binding to an A-site rRNA model oligonucleotide. J Mol Biol. 1996;262:421-36. doi: 10.1006/jmbi.1996.0526.

Recht MI, Douthwaite S, Dahlquist KD, Puglisi JD. Effect of mutations in the A site of 16 S rRNA on aminoglycoside antibiotic-ribosome interaction. J Mol Biol. 1999; 286:33-43. doi: 10.1006/jmbi.1998.2446.

Rowe SM, Varga K, Rab A, Bebok Z, Byram K, Li Y, Sorscher EJ, Clancy JP. Restoration of W1282X CFTR activity by enhanced expression. Am J Respir Cell Mol Biol. 2007;37:347-56. doi: 10.1165/rcmb.2006-0176OC.

Rowe SM, Sloane P, Tang LP, Backer K, Mazur M, Buckley-Lanier J, Nudelman I, Belakhov V, Bebok Z, Schwiebert E, Baasov T, Bedwell DM. Suppression of CFTR premature termination codons and rescue of CFTR protein and function by the synthetic aminoglycoside NB54. J Mol Med (Berl). 2011;89:1149-61. doi: 10.1007/s00109-011-0787-6.

Sako Y, Usuki F, Suga H. A novel therapeutic approach for genetic diseases by introduction of suppressor tRNA. Nucleic Acids Symp Ser (Oxf). 2006;(50):239-40. doi: 10.1093/nass/nrl119.

Schweingruber C, Rufener SC, Zünd D, Yamashita A, Mühlemann O. Nonsense-mediated mRNA decay - mechanisms of substrate mRNA recognition and degradation in mammalian cells. Biochim Biophys Acta. 2013; 1829:612-23. doi: 10.1016/j.bbagrm.2013.02.005.

Sermet-Gaudelus I, Renouil M, Fajac A, Bidou L, Parbaille B, Pierrot S, Davy N, Bismuth E, Reinert P, Lenoir G, Lesure JF, Rousset JP, Edelman A. In vitro prediction of stop-codon suppression by intravenous gentamicin in patients with cystic fibrosis: a pilot study. BMC Med. 2007;5:5. doi: 10.1186/1741-7015-5-5.

Sermet-Gaudelus I, Boeck KD, Casimir GJ, Vermeulen F, Leal T, Mogenet A, Roussel D, Fritsch J, Hanssens L, Hirawat S, Miller NL, Constantine S, Reha A, Ajayi T, Elfring GL, Miller LL. Ataluren (PTC124) induces cystic fibrosis transmembrane conductance regulator protein expression and activity in children with nonsense mutation cystic fibrosis. Am J Respir Crit Care Med. 2010;182: 1262-72. doi: 10.1164/rccm.201001-0137OC.

Sharma J, Du M, Wong E, Mutyam V, Li Y, Chen J, Wangen J, Thrasher K, Fu L, Peng N, Tang L, Liu K, Mathew B, Bostwick RJ, Augelli-Szafran CE, Bihler H, Liang F, Mahiou J, Saltz J, Rab A, Hong J, Sorscher EJ, Mendenhall EM, Coppola CJ, Keeling KM, Green R, Mense M, Suto MJ, Rowe SM, Bedwell DM. A small molecule that induces translational readthrough of CFTR nonsense mutations by eRF1 depletion. Nat Commun. 2021;12:4358. doi: 10.1038/s41467-021-24575-x.

Singh A, Ursic D, Davies J. Phenotypic suppression and misreading *Saccharomyces cerevisiae*. Nature. 1979;277: 146-8. doi: 10.1038/277146a0.

Van de Peer Y, Van den Broeck I, De Rijk P, De Wachter R. Database on the structure of small ribosomal subunit RNA. Nucleic Acids Res. 1994;22:3488-94. doi: 10.1093/nar/22.17.3488.

Vicens Q, Westhof E. Crystal structure of paromomycin docked into the eubacterial ribosomal decoding A site. Structure. 2001;9:647-58. doi: 10.1016/s0969-2126(01)00629-3.

Volkmann K, Lucas JL, Vuga D, Wang X, Brumm D, Stiles C, Kriebel D, Der- Sarkissian A, Krishnan K, Schweitzer C, Liu Z, Malyankar UM, Chiovitti D, Canny M, Durocher D, Sicheri F, Patterson JB. Potent and selective inhibitors of the inositol-requiring enzyme 1 endoribonuclease. J Biol Chem. 2011;286:12743-55. doi: 10.1074/jbc.M110.199737.

Wagner KR, Hamed S, Hadley DW, Gropman AL, Burstein AH, Escolar DM, Hoffman EP, Fischbeck KH. Gentamicin treatment of Duchenne and Becker muscular dystrophy due to nonsense mutations. Ann Neurol. 2001;49:706-11.

Wang D, Zavadil J, Martin L, Parisi F, Friedman E, Levy D, Harding H, Ron D, Gardner LB. Inhibition of nonsense-mediated RNA decay by the tumor microenvironment promotes tumorigenesis. Mol Cell Biol. 2011; 31:3670-80. doi: 10.1128/MCB.05704-11.

Welch EM, Barton ER, Zhuo J, Tomizawa Y, Friesen WJ, Trifillis P, Paushkin S, Patel M, Trotta CR, Hwang S, Wilde RG, Karp G, Takasugi J, Chen G, Jones S, Ren H, Moon YC, Corson D, Turpoff AA, Campbell JA, Conn MM, Khan A, Almstead NG, Hedrick J, Mollin A, Risher N, Weetall M, Yeh S, Branstrom AA, Colacino JM, Babiak J, Ju WD, Hirawat S, Northcutt VJ, Miller LL, Spatrick P, He F, Kawana M, Feng H, Jacobson A, Peltz SW, Sweeney HL. PTC124 targets genetic disorders caused by nonsense mutations. Nature. 2007;447:87-91. doi: 10.1038/nature05756.

Wek RC, Jiang HY, Anthony TG. Coping with stress: eIF2 kinases and translational control. Biochem Soc Trans. 2006;34:7-11. doi: 10.1042/BST20060007.

Wilschanski M, Famini C, Blau H, Rivlin J, Augarten A, Avital A, Kerem B, Kerem E. A pilot study of the effect of gentamicin on nasal potential difference measurements in cystic fibrosis patients carrying stop mutations. Am J Respir Crit Care Med. 2000; 161:860-5. doi: 10.1164/ajrccm.161.3.9904116.

Wilschanski M, Yahav Y, Yaacov Y, Blau H, Bentur L, Rivlin J, Aviram M,Bdolah-Abram T, Bebok Z, Shushi L, Kerem B, Kerem E. Gentamicin-induced correction of CFTR function in patients with cystic fibrosis and CFTR stop mutations. N Engl J Med. 2003;349:1433-41. doi: 10.1056/NEJMoa022170.

Xue X, Mutyam V, Tang L, Biswas S, Du M, Jackson LA, Dai Y, Belakhov V, Shalev M, Chen F, Schacht J, J Bridges R, Baasov T, Hong J, Bedwell DM, Rowe SM. Synthetic aminoglycosides efficiently suppress cystic fibrosis transmembrane conductance regulator nonsense mutations and are enhanced by ivacaftor. Am J Respir Cell Mol Biol. 2014;50:805-16. doi: 10.1165/rcmb.2013-0282OC.

Xue X, Mutyam V, Thakerar A, Mobley J, Bridges RJ, Rowe SM, Keeling KM, Bedwell DM. Identification of the amino acids inserted during suppression of CFTR nonsense mutations and determination of their functional consequences. Hum Mol Genet. 2017;26:3116-3129. doi: 10.1093/hmg/ddx196.

5. CFTR correctors and CFTR potentiators

5.1. Preclinical studies

Burkhard Tümmler

When by 1989 the *CFTR* gene had been identified to be the target of CF-causing mutations (Kerem et al., 1989), the scientific community was initially hoping that within a few years a cure could be provided by gene therapy. However, research of the early 1990s unravelled numerous obstacles, which clarified that it will take decades until gene therapy would become a realistic option for the treatment of CF. More than thirty years later we now finally envisage that we will be able to set up the toolbox of gene editing, somatic stem cells and non-viral vectors for genomic restoration of CF. Considering the bleak perspectives of a genetic cure of CF in the midst 1990s, academia and industry started an alternative strategy for a causative treatment, i.e. to screen for small molecules that reverse the basic defect in CF. Conceptually these envisaged CFTR modulators were classified in either amplifiers, correctors or potentiators.

> Amplifiers enrich ER-associated CFTR mRNA and increase its translational efficiency through increasing the fraction of CFTR mRNA associated with polysomes. Correctors improve the posttranslational processing and trafficking of mutant CFTR and potentiators increase the CFTR-mediated transport of chloride and bicarbonate.

Academic laboratories in the US, Canada, France and Italy set up high-throughput assays to screen libraries of small molecules for anion transport in p.Phe508del *CFTR*-transfected epithelial cells. Hits identified in immortalized cell lines were then verified in primary CF cell cultures and more recently in organotypic culture systems from disease-specific induced pluripotent stem cells (iPSCs; Merkert et al., 2019). By 2005 the screening of 150,000 chemically diverse compounds had already yielded more than 1,500 p.Phe508del-CFTR correctors (aminoarylthiazoles, quinazolinylaminopyrimidinones, and bisaminomethylbithiazoles) with micromolar potency that produced greater apical membrane chloride current than did low-temperature rescue (Pedemonte et al., 2005). Thereafter, the academic labs discovered novel chemical classes of potentiators (Brindani et al., 2020) and correctors (Pesci et al., 2015) including ARN23765 that showed a potency of 38 picomolar in p.Phe508del bronchial epithelial cells, which is more than 5,000-fold lower than any yet clinically approved corrector drug (Pedemonte et al., 2020). Moreover, the researchers identified novel chemical scaffolds that demonstrated synergy with the drug lumacaftor (Boinet et al., 2014; Phuan et al., 2014) and novel potentiators that unlike ivacaftor do not interfere with p.Phe508 CFTR stability or corrector action (Phuan et al., 2015). The database CandActCFTR provides detailed and comprehensive information on these candidate therapeutics for the activation of CFTR-mediated ion conductance aiding systems-biology approaches to identify substances that will synergistically activate CFTR-mediated ion conductance based on published data (Nietert et al., 2021). Despite these impressive achievements, none of these molecules discovered by academia was further developed by safety pharmacology and toxicology and tested in clinical trials. Thus, hereinafter we will focus on the compounds that entered the clinical arena and were finally approved by the regulatory authorities. By 2021, Galapagos/AbbVie and Vertex Pharmaceuticals were the two major research-based pharmaceutical manufacturers that pursue the development of CFTR modulators.

As outlined in the previous chapters of this monograph, a broad pipeline of tools and assays is meanwhile available for the preclinical characterization of potential CFTR modulators. The molecular action of compounds of interest has been studied with the native or recombinant CFTR protein, in recombinant cell lines, organoids, primary cells or CF animals (mouse, rat, ferret, pig). Binding site and mechanism of modulators have been resolved with the reconstituted protein in model membranes and by cryo-electron microscopy. Pulse-chase and proteolysis kinetics, immunoblots and immunocytochemistry provided information about the stability, processing, half-life and spatiotemporal localization of mutant CFTR. CFTR function as an ion channel was examined by halide efflux assays in cell culture, the measurement of

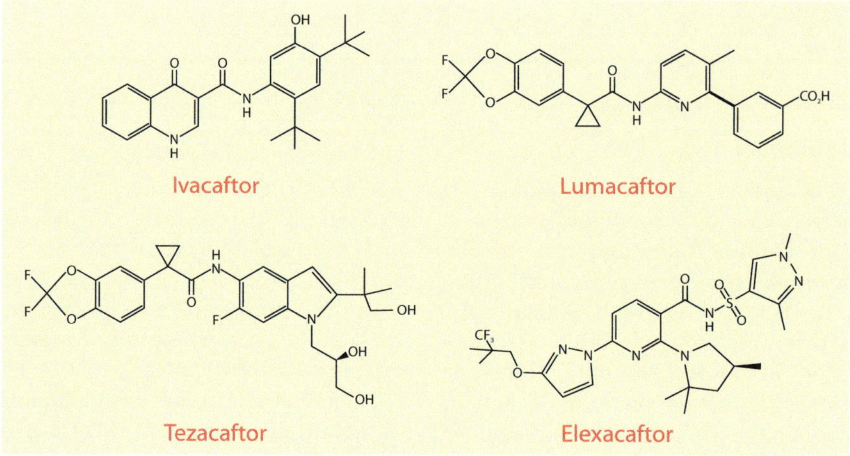

Figure 5.1: Chemical structure of approved CFTR modulators.

ion flow across epithelia in Ussing chambers and the assessment of properties of the ion channel in patch clamp experiments.

Ivacaftor

The yet most thoroughly characterized compound is the CFTR potentiator ivacaftor (IVA, VX-770, IUPAC name: N-(2,4-di-tert-butyl-5-hydroxyphenyl)-4-oxo-1,4-dihydroquinoline-3-carboxamide; ☞ Figure 5.1; van Goor et al., 2009). The opening of the CFTR ion channel normally requires the binding and subsequent hydrolysis of ATP. In contrast, picomolar ivacaftor reversibly enhances ATP-independent opening of the channel and thereby overcomes the defective ATP-dependent opening of CF-causing gating mutations (Eckford et al., 2012; Jih and Hwang, 2013; Csanády and Töröcsik, 2019). CFTR open probability increases by stabilizing pre-hydrolytic states with respect to closed states (Kopeikin et al., 2014; Langron et al., 2018). If CFTR was solubilized with detergents, ivacaftor bound to CFTR at the protein-lipid interface, docking into a cleft formed by transmembrane helices 4, 5, and 8 (Liu et al., 2019). These cryo electron microscopy data contradicted mass spectrometric findings of hydrogen/deuterium exchange, which assigned the binding site of ivacaftor to the intracellular loop 4 (Byrnes et al., 2018). A more recent photoaffinity labelling study of native CFTR in phospholipid membranes confirmed the intracellular loop 4 as the major binding site for ivacaftor and the region previously identified by cryo-EM as the second minor binding site of CFTR (Laselva et al., 2021). In summary, ivacaftor stabilizes the channel open configuration by binding to the intracellular loop 4 that connects the nucleotide binding domains to the conduction path of the CFTR channel.

Ivacaftor shows some actions not expected from a CFTR modulator. First, it structurally resembles quinolone antibiotics and indeed confers moderate antibacterial activity against the typical CF pathogens *Staphylococcus aureus* and *Pseudomonas aeruginosa* (Reznikov et al., 2014). Second, ivacaftor persists much longer in its target cells than estimated from serum pharmacokinetics, which may lead to overdosage and attenuation of efficacy (Guhr Lee et al., 2020). Third, the lipophilic molecule modifies the fluidity and organization of lipid bilayers (Chin et al., 2018), which may explain why chronic exposure to ivacaftor destabilizes mutant CFTR in the plasma membrane that has been rescued with a CFTR corrector (Cholon et al., 2014; Veit et al., 2015; 2020; Becq et al., 2021).

Animal models are informative for understanding the pathogenesis and progression of CF. At present, we still do not know at what age CFTR modulation can be safely initiated. Theoretically, the earliest time point of therapy should be that which provides the most benefit for an inherited condition such as cystic fibrosis. Experiments in a p.Gly 551Asp ferret CF model (Sun et al., 2019) suggest that CFTR is important for establishing organ function early in life. In utero and postnatal administration of a CFTR modulator provided partial protection from developmental pathologies in the pancreas, intestine, and male reproductive tract and the typical symptoms of cystic fibrosis, but drug withdrawal led to the rapid re-establishment of disease. However, ivacaftor may not prevent all pathologies caused by defective gating of CFTR. Administration of ivacaftor to a humanized h-p.Gly551Asp rat model reduced the concentration of cytokines in the lung in the absence of an inflammatory stimulus, but was less effective in inflamed tissue indicating that CFTR activation is not enough to resolve inflammation in the airways (Green et al., 2021).

Although there are more than 2,000 known sequence variants in *CFTR*, the vast majority of CF is homozygous or compound heterozygous for the most common mutation p.Phe508del. Phe508del CFTR protein is defective in posttranslational processing and trafficking. Newly synthesized Phe508del CFTR fails to adopt a wild-type fold in the ER, is targeted to ER-associated degradation and is removed faster from the apical membrane by endocytosis. Consequently, p.Phe508del homozygous subjects express only low amounts of complex-glycosylated Phe508del CFTR and low or no residual Phe508del CFTR-mediated chloride and bicarbonate secretory activity. Attenuation of the translational elongation rate by the knock-down of components of the ribosomal stalk increases the folding efficiency as well as the conformational stability of the Phe508del CFTR (Veit et al., 2016; Oliver et al., 2019). However, small molecules turned out to be more efficient and more practicable to improve the folding of Phe508del CFTR. The analysis of second-site suppressor mutations revealed that a robust correction of the conformational defects of Phe508del CFTR requires the stabilization of the interfaces between the two nucleotide binding domains (NBDs) and the membrane-spanning domains (type I) and the stabilization of nucleotide binding domains 2 (NBD2, type II) and Phe508del NBD1 (type III; Okiyoneda et al., 2013). Combinations of type I, II and III correctors restored 50-100% of wild-type-level Phe508del CFTR biogenesis and stability in immortalized and primary human airway epithelia (Veit et al., 2018). Concomitantly, the correctors decrease mucus concentration, relax mucus network ultrastructure, improve mucus transport and change the cellular lipidome, in particular make the epithelial cells less susceptible to apoptosis by reducing the levels of ceramide (Gardner et al., 2020; Liessi et al., 2020; Morrison et al., 2021; Veltman et al., 2021).

Lumacaftor

Lumacaftor (LUM, VX-809, IUPAC name: 3-[6-[[[1-(2,2-difluoro-1,3-benzodioxol-5-yl)cyclopropyl] carbonyl] amino]-3-methyl-2-pyridinyl]-benzoic acid; ☞ Figure 5.1) has been the first CFTR corrector approved for use in humans (van Goor et al., 2011). This type I corrector acts early during CFTR biosynthesis (Loo and Clarke, 2017; Kleizen et al., 2021) so that Phe508del CFTR can exit the ER. It improves the co-translational folding of transmembrane domain 1 (TMD1). The subsequent early post-translational TMD1:NBD1 packing facilitates the most critical step of Phe508del CFTR folding, i.e. the binding to cytoplasmic loop 4 (ICL4), leading to progression of domain assembly in the absence of folded Phe508del-NBD1 (Kleizen et al., 2021). Further allosteric effects of lumacaftor are the stabilization of the NBD1:ICL4 and NBD1:ICL1 interfaces, of the transmembrane helices 3 and 4 and of the TMD1:TMD2 interaction (Farinha et al., 2013; He et al., 2013; Ren et al., 2013; Hudson et al., 2017; Loo and Clarke, 2017; Laselva et al., 2018; Krainer et al., 2020).

Tezacaftor

Tezacaftor (TEZ, VX-661, IUPAC name: (R)-1-(2,2-difluorobenzo[d][1,3]dioxol-5-yl)-N-(1-(2,3-dihydroxypropyl)-6-fluoro-2-(1-hydroxy-2-methylpropan-2-yl)-1H-indol-5-yl)cyclopropane carboxamide; ☞ Figure 5.1) has been the second type I corrector that has been approved for the treatment of people with CF with one or two p.Phe508del alleles. Immunoblotting and in silico docking experiments proposed a similar composite multi-domain binding pocket for lumacaftor and tezacaftor comprised of residues within the NBD1: ICL4 interface (Molinski et al., 2018).

Two type III correctors have so far been compared in combination therapy with tezacaftor and ivacaftor, i.e. bumacaftor (VX-659, IUPAC name: *N*-(benzenesulfonyl)-6-[3-[2-[1-(trifluoromethyl) cyclopropyl]ethoxy]pyrazol-1-yl]-2-[(4*S*)-2,2,4-trimethylpyrrolidin-1-yl]pyridine-3-carboxamide) and elexacaftor (ELX, VX-445, IUPAC name: *N*-(1,3-dimethylpyrazol-4-yl)sulfonyl-6-[3-(3,3,3-trifluoro-2,2-dimethylpropoxy)pyrazol-1-yl]-2-[(4*S*)-2,2,4-trimethylpyrrolidin-1-yl] pyridine-3-carboxamide; ☞ Figure 5.1). Elexacaftor synergistically restores Phe508del CFTR processing in combination with type I or II correctors (Veit et al., 2020; Becq et al., 2021) and moreover acts as a co-potentiator of Phe508del, Gly551Asp and Met1101Lys CFTR chloride channels (Laselva et al., 2021; Shaughnessy et al., 2021; Veit et al., 2021). Exposure of primary Phe508del homozygous epithelia to a triple combination of ELX/TEZ/IVA restored Phe508del CFTR chloride channel function to about 60% of wild-type levels (Veit et al., 2020; Capurro et al., 2021). However, when Phe508del homozygous cells were treated with ivacaftor combined to any correctors (LUM or TEZ or ELX), the Phe508del CFTR current was unresponsive to the subsequent acute addition of ivacaftor (Cholon et al., 2014; Veit et al., 2014; 2020; Becq et al., 2021). Ivacaftor diminished the folding efficiency and the metabolic stability of Phe508 CFTR at the ER and post-ER compartments and destabilized rescued Phe508del CFTR at the plasma membrane causing reduced cell surface Phe508 CFTR density and function. This dose-dependent reversal of Phe508del CFTR rescue has not been observed with the CFTR potentiators GLPG/ABBV-1837 and GLPG/ABBV-2451 in conjunction with the CFTR Corrector ABBV-2222/GLPG2222 (Gees et al., 2018; Wang et al., 2018; Singh et al., 2020; van der Plas et al., 2021).

Meanwhile close to 2,000 disease-causing variants are known in the *CFTR* gene, the majority of which are rare or so far known in only a single family. To make CFTR modulator therapy available to almost all patients who carry at least one allele with a responsive mutation to CFTR modulation, one needs reliable *in vitro* systems that can be benchmarked against wild-type and the most common genotypes. Thus, academia and industry set up a pipeline of standardized recombinant cell lines (Yu et al., 2012; Sosnay et al., 2013; van Goor et al., 2014; Han et al., 2018) and nasal and rectal organoid cultures (Dekkers et al., 2013; 2016a; 2016b; Anderson et al., 2021; de Poel et al., 2021; Ramalho et al., 2021) to compare residual CFTR function and drug-modulated CFTR function of a large collection of *CFTR* mutations and genotypes. The responses of the organoids to drug therapy depended on both the *CFTR* mutation and the genetic background of the subjects, which may partly explain the broad Gaussian distribution of clinical efficacy seen among study participants in clinical trials (Dekkers et al., 2016a). The swelling activity of nasal organoids paralleled the patient's clinical response to monotherapy with ivacaftor and triple therapy with ELX/TEZ/IVA suggesting that this bioassay may predict the individual patient's response to a modulator drug (Anderson et al., 2021).

Panels of cell lines engineered to express CFTR mutants led to more robust and reproducible comparisons of mutant phenotype, but this standardization on one cell line and genetic background will of course not capture the genetic and environmental modifiers of the processing and function of mutated CFTR. Han and colleagues (2018) examined variants that represent 87% of individuals in the CFTR2 database with at least 1 missense variant. The magnitude of drug response to IVA, LUM or IVA-LUM combination was highly correlated with residual CFTR function in both recombinant human CF bronchial epithelial (CFBE41o-) and Fischer rat thyroid (FRT) cells. These consistent findings may have led to FDA's seminal decision that ELX/TEZ/IVA triple therapy is indicated for the treatment of CF in patients who have at least one mutation in the *CFTR* gene that is responsive based on *in vitro* data.

5.2. Clinical pharmacology: Pharmacokinetics, metabolism and drug-drug interactions

Martin Hug

5.2.1. Polypharmacy and Cystic Fibrosis

Over the past 80 years, advances in medicine have increased CF patient's quality and expectancy. Significant impact was caused by modulators of the disease causing Cystic Fibrosis Transmembrane Conductance Regulator (CFTR) protein (Gramegna et al., 2020). This causal therapeutic approach has improved the prognosis but did not entirely cure the underlying disease. Most patients will still depend on routine treatments. Comorbidities as well as acute exacerbations may result in additional therapeutic interventions. Prior to the introduction of the CFTR modulators a survey among 204 CF patients estimated a median number of seven different drugs that were used on a daily basis (Sawicki et al., 2013). A more recent publication determined an even higher number of 10 (6-15) therapeutic measures (Davies et al., 2020). It is no surprise that under such conditions drug-drug interactions are almost inevitable. At the same time the risk for adverse events, which not only stipulate the therapeutic goal but also have a negative impact on the patient's adherence, is increased.

5.2.2. Comparison of the CFTR modulators

During the past 10 years, four CFTR Modulators have received marketing approval. Despite their somewhat different mode of action all these compounds are highly lipophilic and strongly bind to plasma proteins (Tsai et al., 2020). This results in a relatively prolonged terminal half-life and bears the risk that in the case of adverse events rapid withdrawal of the substances is almost impossible. To this end, the profile of side-effects of the CFTR modulators appears to be benign and is hardly discernable from the symptoms caused by the underlying disease (Gavioli et al., 2021). Data derived from preclinical and clinical trials indicate that ivacaftor increases the risk for cataracts which is why the manufacturer recommends regular controls of the visual acuity (Talamo Guevara and McColley, 2017). For the combination of luma- and ivacaftor (Orkambi®) symptoms such as shortness of breath and chest discomfort have been reported (Burgel et al., 2020). Little to nothing is known about the root cause of these symptoms. A common feature of all CFTR modulators is a temporal or permanent increase in liver enzymes. This is relevant with respect to drug-drug interactions.

5.2.3. Pharmacokinetics of the CFTR modulators

The mechanisms through which adverse events occur can be divided into pharmacokinetic and pharmacodynamic interactions. In the case of the CFTR modulators the former is of higher clinical relevance. The pharmacokinetics of any drug can best be described with the LADME model. As depicted in Table 5.1, any given drug must cross several barriers until it reaches its target. At the same time several mechanisms are in place to eliminate the substance from the body. Since all currently approved CFTR modulators are administered orally, the liberation is the first challenge for their uptake. Solid drugs disintegrate in the upper gastrointestinal tract. Therefore, enough liquid is essential which needs to be communicated to the patients and their caregivers. The CFTR modulators are very lipophilic and almost insoluble in water. To ensure sufficient resorption, solubilisation is required. The summary of product characteristics (SMPC) of Kalydeco®, Orkambi®, Symkevi® and Kaftrio®/Trikafta® recommend that the tablets should be taken with food that is high in fat. This measure may increase the absorption by a factor 2.5-4.

5.2.3.1. Distribution

An important pharmacokinetic parameter is the apparent volume of distribution (Vd). The magnitude of Vd largely depends on the binding of the respective drug to plasma proteins. Due to the physical-chemical properties of the CFTR modulators, Vd is relatively high. Table 5.1 reports the proportion of the active substance bound to plasma proteins. CF patients often suffer from a latent or acute deficiency in plasma proteins which may cause larger fluctuations in free serum levels of drugs than in the healthy population. To this end it is unclear whether CFTR modulators compete with other active substances for the binding sites of the plasma proteins, which in turn may have an impact on the total bioavailability (Schneider et al., 2015).

	Ivacaftor	Lumacaftor	Tezacaftor	Elexacaftor
L(iberation)	oral	oral	oral	oral
A(bsorption)	intestinal	intestinal	intestinal	intestinal
D(istribution)	PPB: 99%	PPB: 99%	PPB: 99%	PPB: 99%
M(etabolism)	hepatic	hepatic	hepatic	hepatic
E(limination)	feces: 87.8%	feces: 51%	feces: 72%, renal: 14%	feces: 87.3%, renal: 0.2%
$T_{1/2}$	12h	26h	67h	25h

Table 5.1: Pharmacokinetic properties of CFTR modulators. PPB = plasma protein binding.

5.2.3.2. Metabolism

Active pharmaceutical substances are often referred to as xenobiotics that our body is perfectly equipped to detoxify. The main goal is to turn lipophilic molecules into water-soluble degradation products. Most of these processes occur in the liver and can be divided into phase-1 and phase-2 reactions. During the first phase the molecule is oxidized while the second phase is characterized by conjugation of the reaction product with hydrophilic residues such as glucuronic or sulfuric acid. In most cases this process is accompanied by a partial or complete loss in pharmacologic activity. The phase-1 reaction is triggered by the activity of an assortment of cytochrome P-450 enzymes (Cyp-450). To this end, more than 50 different isoforms of this enzyme complex are known (McLean and Munro, 2018). Within this group, eight play a role in drug metabolism. These have a different specificity for the respective active substance (Indiana University School of Medicine & Division of Clinical Pharmacology, o. J.). All CFTR modulators are substrates of the Cyp-450 system. Due to the historical development, a body of evidence has already been collected for ivacaftor (Kalydeco®), which was approved in 2012. The main metabolites hydroxymethyl-ivacaftor (M1) und ivacaftor-carboxylate (M6) are caused by the activity of the Cyp 3A457 Isoform (Vonk et al., 2021). In subsequent steps the molecules are transformed by glucuronidations into the metabolites M3, M7 and M8, respectively. It does not surprise that during the simultaneous administration of several substances metabolized by Cyp 3A457 competition among the same target may occur. It is a known fact that some substances not only serve as a substrate of the Cyp-450 system but moreover increase the activity of these enzymes. Such molecules are referred to as inducers. Other compounds have the opposite effect and inhibit enzyme activity, which is why they are called inhibitors (Mc Lean and Munro, 2018; Indiana University School of Medicine & Division of Clinical Pharmacology, o. J.). Using publicly available databases, estimates on the impact of Cyp-inhibitors or inducers with substrates of the respective enzymes can be made (Estimation of the variation of exposure due to a drug-drug interaction—DDI-Predictor Academic version, o. J.).

5.2.4. Impact of Cyp-inhibitors on ivacaftor serum levels

Among the great many inhibitors of the Cyp 3A457 enzyme complex are not only food products such as citrus fruits but also substances that may be used as co-medication in CF patients. Of particular interest are antibacterial and antimycotic agents. The simultaneous administration of such substances may potentially increase the serum concentration of ivacaftor by a factor of 5-10. Table 5.2 lists the effects of several antimicrobial substances on the area under curve of ivacaftor (modelled after Estimation of the variation of exposure due to a drug-drug interaction—DDI-Predictor Academic version, o. J.). The SMPC of all drugs that contain ivacaftor recommend dose reduction in such a case.

Drug	Estimated increase in $AUC_{Ivacaftor}$
Azithromycin	1.11 (0.83 - 1.48)
Ciprofloxacin	1 (0.76 - 1.32)
Roxithromycin	1.46 (1.02 - 2.06)
Erythromycin	3.82 (2.1 - 6.96)
Clarithromycin	4.81 (2.55 - 9.07)
Isavuconazol	2.02 (1.28 - 3.19)
Posaconazol	3.84 (2.11 - 7)
Fluconazol	4.26 (2.3 - 7.9)
Itraconazol	6.9 (3.51 - 13.56)
Voriconazol	8.47 (4.24 - 16.94)

Table 5.2: Effect of CYP 3A4/5/7 inhibitors area under curve (AUC) of ivacaftor. Data from https://www.ddi-predictor.org/predictor/ddi.

5.2.5. Impact of liver function

A significant fraction of drug metabolism occurs in the liver. Impaired function of this organ affects the pharmacokinetics of most drugs. Unfortunately up to 40% of all CF patients develop pathological changes of the liver that impacts mortality in 2-5% of all cases (Sakiani et al., 2019). The degree of liver damage is classified by the Child-Pugh-Score (CPS; Pugh et al., 1973). Even at the lowest CPS (A) an increase in ivacaftor AUC can be expected. In such cases, dose adjustments can be recommended whereas at the most severe CPS C treatment should be suspended according to the SMPC.

5.2.6. Inducers of the Cyp-System

Several chemical but also plant derived substances have the potential to increase the activity of the Cyp-system. This results in the accelerated degradation of the substrates of the respective isoenzyme. This is particularly pronounced when the ansamycin drugs rifampicin and rifabutin are used. These bactericidal antibiotics are used in CF patients when infections with mycobacteria are suspected or diagnosed. A concomitant treatment with CFTR modulators might lead to lower serum concentrations and subsequently to therapeutic failure. The SMPC of the respective drugs advice against the simultaneous use of Cyp-inducers and CFTR modulators. Interestingly, lumacaftor is not only substrate but also inducer of the Cyp 3A457 isoenzymes. To compensate for the potentially increased metabolism by this substance, the daily recommended dose of ivacaftor is increased by 67% when combined with lumacaftor. Table 5.3 shows the effects of several Cyp-inducers on the AUC of ivacaftor. Clearly, the impact of lumacaftor on drug metabolism is not restricted to ivacaftor. Several other substrates undergo the same fate during simultaneous administration. This is of relevance when CF patients use steroids. Table 5.4 models the potential consequences when lumacaftor is combined with a selection of other active pharmaceutical compounds.

Drug	Estimated decrease in $AUC_{Ivacaftor}$
St. John's Wort	0.48 (0.3 - 0.7)
Rifabutin	0.34 (0.2 - 0.59)
Rifampicin	0.13 (0.07 - 0.26)
Lumacaftor	0.2 (0.11 - 0.38)

Table 5.3: Effect of CYP 3A4/5/7 Inducers. Data from https://www.ddi-predictor.org/predictor/ddi.

Drug	Estimated decrease in AUC_{Drug}
Prednisolone	0.56 (0.37 - 0.85)
Ethinylestradiol	0.46 (0.29 - 0.74)
Dienogest	0.27 (0.15 - 0.49)
Methylprednisolone	0.25 (0.14 - 0.46)
Dexamethason	0.24 (0.13 - 0.44)
Midazolam	0.2 (0.11 - 0.38)

Table 5.4: Effect of lumacaftor on drugs that are used in CF patients. Data from https://www.ddi-predictor.org/predictor/ddi.

5.2.7. Tezacaftor and elexacaftor – novel agents with lower risk for interactions

Due to lumacaftor's significant risk for interactions, the manufacturer of Orkambi® tried to identify other substances that increase CFTR function. The candidate compound tezacaftor is also metabolized by Cyp 3A457. As shown for the other CFTR modulators, simultaneous administration of Cyp 3A457-inhibitors will slow down degradation of tezacaftor whereas inducers will result in the opposite. Preclinical studies in human hepatocytes and recombinant Cyp-450 enzyme preparations showed that tezacaftor has no relevant impact on the metabolic activity. This could subsequently be confirmed by *in vivo* experiments (Garg et al., 2019), which eventually resulted in the development of Symkevi®. Table 5.5 shows the interaction profile of this drug.

Drug	Estimated decrease in AUC_{Drug}
Norethisteron	1.05 (0.98 - 1.12)
Ethinylestradiol	1.12 (1.03 - 1.22)
Midazolam	1.12 (1.01 - 1.25)
Digoxin	1.3 (1.17 - 1.45)

Table 5.5: Effect of tezacaftor on CYP substrates. Data from https://www.ddi-predictor.org/predictor/ddi.

Shortly after Symkevi® had been introduced on the market, combinations of ivacaftor, tezacaftor and yet another substance were studied. The rationale behind this approach was that tezacaftor showed fewer interactions compared with lumacaftor but also demonstrated a lower activity. This dilemma could be overcome by the addition of elexacaftor. But what are the metabolic consequences of such a triple combination? As shown for the other compounds, elexacaftor also undergoes phase-1 modifications. Therefore, interactions with Cyp-inducers and inhibitors are to be expected. In addition, both the parent compound and its main metabolite M23-Elx demonstrate inhibition of the organic anion transporters OATP1 and OATP3. These proteins are expressed in hepatocytes and renal tubules (Smith et al., 2005). Several pharmaceutical substances such as statins and antidiabetic sulfonylurea compounds are taken up into the liver cell by these transporters. In the kidney OAT proteins facilitate the elimination of xenobiotics. This is the reason why the SMPC of Kaftrio®/ Trikafta® advise for increased awareness when substrates of OATP transporters are taken concomitantly. Both elexacaftor and ivacaftor inhibit the Breast Cancer Resistance Protein (BCRP, ABCG2) which eliminates several active substances across intestinal epithelia (Jani et al., 2014). To this end, it is unclear whether interactions with OATP1, OATP3 or BRCP play a clinically relevant role in the treatment of CF patients. Nevertheless, this finding underscores the complex interplay between the CFTR modulators and other drugs.

5.3. Clinical trials

Burkhard Tümmler

Clinical trials on CFTR potentiators and CFTR modulators started in the early years of the millennium. Table 5.6 lists the more than 80 phase 2 and phase 3 studies from the 2005 – 2022 time period and Table 5.7 summarizes the outcome of the major randomized, double-blind, placebo-controlled or active comparator-controlled phase 3 studies. The phase 3 studies typically recruited CF patients with moderately reduced lung function indicated by a FEV1 of 40-90% predicted. Patients within this intermediate range of lung disease are most appropriate to show a sensitive and robust response to CFTR modulation without the risk of severe adverse advents due to the medication and without a high frequency of pulmonary exacerbations that are typical for the more severely affected patients with FEV1 less than 40% predicted. The primary endpoint of most studies was the change of FEV1% in absolute percentage points. Other common secondary endpoints were the change in body weight and in the frequency of pulmonary exacerbations, the change in the quality of life assessed by the Cystic Fibrosis Questionnaire-Revised respiratory domain score (Quittner et al., 2005) and the change in sweat chloride concentration as a measure of the reversion of the basic defect.

Clinical drug development was similar for the various compounds. Ivacaftor, the first oral drug that made it to the clinic may be taken as an illustration of the long journey from the first tests in humans until the examination of the most vulnerable groups, i.e. infants and pregnant women. The six phase 1 studies in healthy male adults investigated formulations, pharmacokinetics of drug and its metabolites, routes and extent of elimination, potential drug-drug interactions and safety and tolerability of multiple and/or escalating doses. The first phase 2 study (Accurso et al., 2010) randomly assigned 39 adults with CF and at least one p.Gly551Asp *CFTR* allele to receive oral ivacaftor every 12 hours at a dose of 25, 75, or 150 mg or placebo for 14 days (in part 1 of the study) or ivacaftor every 12 hours at a dose of 150 or 250 mg or placebo for 28 days (in part 2 of the study). At day 28, the cumulative depolarization response of CFTR-mediated chloride conductance in the NPD had significantly increased and the chloride concentration in the sweat test had dropped from values in the classical CF range of about 100 mmol/L to the borderline or even normal range. Two subsequent 24-week or 48-week phase 3 studies in large cohorts of children (Davies et al., 2013a), adolescents and adults (Ramsey et al., 2011) uncovered that this modulation of the basic defect was accompanied by significant clinical improvements. Within the first four weeks of treatment, the study participants gained 10 percentage points of FEV1, which was maintained during the study period. The risk of pulmonary exacerbations was significantly reduced by 55%. Anthropometry improved which was particularly prominent in children and adolescents.

Next, the clinical response to ivacaftor was examined in p.Gly551Asp homozygous or compound heterozygous CF children elder than 6 years with preserved spirometry of more than 90% FEV1 predicted, but an abnormal lung clearance index (LCI) as a measure of ventilation inhomogeneity (Davies et al., 2013b). During treatment with ivacaftor, the LCI dropped significantly compared to placebo implying mucus retention in the small airways could be resolved by the correction of the basic defect with ivacaftor. This data provided the first evidence that mutation-specific therapy should be started early during the clinically asymptomatic stage of CF lung disease.

Subsequent trials showed the efficacy and safety of ivacaftor for CF carriers of non-p.Gly551Asp gating mutations (De Boeck et al., 2014) including p.Arg117His (Moss et al., 2015) the latter being only slightly defective in both channel gating and

Study	Phase	*CFTR* mutation genotype	Age (yr)	Follow-up	Reference
A. Monotherapy with potentiator ivacaftor					
VX06-770-101	2	hetero- or homozygous for p.Gly551Asp	≥18	28 days	Accurso et al. N Engl J Med 2010;363:1991-2003
VX08-770-102 (STRIVE)	3	hetero- or homozygous for p.Gly551Asp	≥12	48 weeks	Ramsey et al. N Engl J Med 2011;365:1663-72
VX08-770-103 (ENVISION)	3	hetero- or homozygous for p.Gly551Asp	6-11	48 weeks	Davies et al. Am J Respir Crit Care Med 2013;187: 1219-25
VX-770-105 (PERSIST)	3	hetero- or homozygous for p.Gly551Asp	≥ 6	96 weeks	McKone et al. Lancet Respir Med 2014;2:902-10
NCT01262352	2	hetero- or homozygous for p.Gly551Asp	≥ 6	84 days	Davies et al. Lancet Respir Med 2013;1:630-8
VX-770-108 (KIWI)	3	hetero- or homozygous for p.Gly551Asp	2-5	24 weeks	Davies et al. Lancet Respir Med 2016;4:107-15.
VX-770-109 (KLIMB)	3	hetero- or homozygous for p.Gly551Asp	2-5	88 weeks	Rosenfeld et al. J Cyst Fibros 2019;18:838-43
VX-770-110 (KONDUCT)	3	hetero- or homozygous for p.Arg117His	≥ 6	28 weeks	Moss et al. Lancet Respir Med 2015;3:524-33
VX-770-111 (KONNECTION)	3	carrier of at least one non-p.Gly551Asp gating mutation	≥ 6	40 weeks	De Boeck et al. J Cyst Fibros 2014;13:674-80
NCT01521338	3	carrier of non-p.Gly551Asp gating mutation	≥ 6	6 months	Guimbellot et al. J Cyst Fibros 2019;18:102-9
VX-770-112	3	Roll-over from 110 or 111	≥ 6	108 weeks	
VX-770-113; NCT01685801	N-of-1	mutations conferring residual function	≥ 12	16 weeks	Nick et al. J Cyst Fibros 2020;19:91-8.
NCT02725567 ARRIVAL	3	carrier of at least one gating mutation	1-2	24 weeks	Rosenfeld et al. Lancet Respir Med 2018;6:545-53
NCT02725567 ARRIVAL	3	carrier of at least one gating mutation	0-1	24 weeks	Davies et al. Am J Respir Crit Care Med 2021;203:585-93
VX-15-770-124	3	carrier of at least one gating mutation	< 1	34 weeks	
VX-770-126	3	carrier of at least one gating mutation	< 2	128 weeks	
NCT01784419	N-of-1	PS genotypes; exclusions: homozygous for p.Phe508 del, carrier of gating mutation	≥ 16	6 weeks	McGarry et al. Pediatr Pulmonol 2017;52:472-79
NCT01937325	4	hetero- or homozygous for p.Gly551Asp	≥ 16	3 months	Edgeworth et al. Clin Sci (Lond) 2017;131:2037-45
	4	hetero- or homozygous for p.Gly551Asp	≥ 16	6 months	King et al., Nutrition 2021;85:111124
NCT02142464	4	hetero- or homozygous for p.Gly551Asp	≥ 5	3 months	Stallings et al. J Pediatr 2018;201:229-37
NCT01707290	3	participants of 110, 111, 113 studies	≥ 6	104 weeks	Pilewski et al. Pulm Ther 2020;6:303-13
NCT 01521338	4	hetero- or homozygous for p.Gly551Asp	≥ 6	3 months	Donaldson et al. JCI Insight 2018;3:e122695

Study	Phase	*CFTR* mutation genotype	Age (yr)	Follow-up	Reference
Vertex770-104 (DISCOVER)	2	homozygous for p.Phe508del	≥ 12	22 weeks	Flume et al. Chest 2012;142: 718-24
B. Monotherapy with potentiator GLPG1837					
NCT02707562 (SAPHIRA1)	2	hetero- or homozygous for p.Gly551Asp	≥ 18	4 weeks	Davies et al. J Cyst Fibros 2019;18:693-9
C. Monotherapy with cavosonstat (N91115), an inhibitor of S-nitrosoglutathione reductase					
NCT02275936, NCT02013388	1	homozygous for p.Phe508del	≥ 18	28 days	Donaldson et al. J Cyst Fibros 2017;16:371-9
D. Monotherapy with riociguat, a guanylate cyclase stimulator					
NCT02170025	2	homozygous for p.Phe508del	≥ 18	28 days	Derichs et al. J Cyst Fibros 2021:S1569-1993(21)01329-1
E. Monotherapy with potentiator VX-561					
VX-561-101	2	hetero- or homozygous for gating mutation	≥ 18	16 weeks	
F. Monotherapy with QR-010 (antisense oligonucleotide eluforsen)					
ProQR PQ-010-001	1	homozygous for p.Phe508del	≥ 18	8 weeks	Drevinek et al. J Cyst Fibros 2020;19:99-107
ProQR PQ-10-002	1	hetero- or homozygous for p.Phe508del	≥ 18	7 weeks	Sermet-Gaudelus et al. J Cyst Fibros 2019;18:536-42
G. Monotherapy with potentiator PTI-808					
PTI-801-01	1 / 2	homozygous for p.Phe508del	≥ 18	30 days	
H. Monotherapy with lumacaftor					
VX08-809-101	2	homozygous for p.Phe508del	≥ 18	28 days	Clancy et al. Thorax 2012;67:12-8
I. Combination therapy with corrector lumacaftor and potentiator ivacaftor					
VX-809-102	2	hetero- or homozygous for p.Phe508del	≥ 18	2 months	Boyle et al. Lancet Respir Med 2014;2:527-38
VX-809-103 (TRAFFIC)	3	homozygous for p.Phe508del	≥ 12	24 weeks	Wainwright et al. N Engl J Med 2015;373:220-31
VX-809-104 (TRANSPORT)	3	homozygous for p.Phe508del	≥ 12	24 weeks	Wainwright et al. N Engl J Med 2015;373:220-31
VX-809-105 (PROGRESS)	3	homozygous for p.Phe508del	≥ 12	96 weeks	Konstan et al. Lancet Respir Med 2017;5:107-18
VX-809-106	3	homozygous for p.Phe508del	≥ 12	52 weeks	Taylor-Cousar et al. J Cyst Fibros 2018;17:228-35
VX13-809-011b	3	homozygous for p.Phe508del	6-11	27 weeks	Milla et al. Am J Respir Crit Care Med 2017;195:912-20
VX-809-109	3	homozygous for p.Phe508del	6-11	24 weeks	Ratjen et al. Lancet Respir Med 2017;5:557-67
VX-809-110	3	homozygous for p.Phe508del	6-11	96 weeks	Chilvers et al. Lancet Respir Med 2021;9:721-32
VX15-809-115	3	homozygous for p.Phe508del	2-5	24 weeks	McNamara et al. Lancet Respir Med 2019;7:325-335
VX16-809-116	3	homozygous for p.Phe508del	2-5	96 weeks	Hoppe et al. Lancet Respir Med 2021;9:977-88
VX16-809-121	3	homozygous for p.Phe508del	2-5	96 weeks	DZL Consortium
VX-16-809-122 Part A	3	homozygous for p.Phe508del	1-2	35 days	

Study	Phase	*CFTR* mutation genotype	Age (yr)	Follow-up	Reference
VX-16-809-122 Part B	3	homozygous for p.Phe508del	1-2	38 weeks	
NCT02807415	4	homozygous for p.Phe508del	≥ 12	16 weeks	Graeber et al. a: Am J Respir Crit Care Med 2018;197: 1433-42; b: Ann Am Thorac Soc 2021;18:971-80
NCT02965326	4	homozygous for p.Phe508del	≥ 12	6 months	Pranke et al. Am J Respir Crit Care Med 2019;199: 123-26
NCT02477319	4	homozygous for p.Phe508del	≥ 6	12 months	Sagel et al. Ann Am Thorac Soc 2021;18:75-83
J. Combination therapy with corrector tezacaftor and potentiator ivacaftor					
VX-661-101	2	homozygous for p.Phe508del or compound heterozygous p.Phe508del/p.Gly551Asp	≥ 18 or ≥ 12 (for the hetero-zygous)	84 days	Donaldson et al. Am J Respir Crit Care Med 2018;197: 214-24
VX-661-103	2	homozygous for p.Phe508del	≥ 18	20 weeks	
VX-661-106 (EVOLVE)	3	homozygous for p.Phe508del	≥ 12	24 weeks	Taylor-Cousar et al. N Engl J Med 2017;377:2013-23
VX-661-107	3	compound heterozygous for p.Phe508del and a minimal function mutation	≥ 12	20 weeks	Munck et al. J Cyst Fibros 2020;19:962-68
VX-661-108 (EXPAND)	3	compound heterozygous for p.Phe508del and a residual-function-mutation	≥ 12	33 weeks	Rowe et al. N Engl J Med 2017;377:2024-35
VX-661-109	3	compound heterozygous for p.Phe508del and a gating mutation	≥ 12	13 weeks	McKone et al. J Cyst Fibros 2021; 20:234-42
VX14-661-110 (EXTEND)	3	homozygous for p.Phe508del or compound heterozygous for p.Phe508del and a resid-ual-function-mutation	≥ 12	96 weeks	Flume et al. Lancet Respir Med 2021;9:733-46
VX-661-111	2	homozygous for p.Phe508del	≥ 18	60 days	
VX15-661-113	3	homozygous for p.Phe508del or compound heterozygous for p.Phe508del and a resid-ual-function-mutation	6-11	24 weeks	Walker et al. J Cyst Fibros 2019;18:708-13
VX-16-661-114	3	homozygous for p.Phe508del	≥12	84 days	Schwarz et al. J Cyst Fibros 2021;20:228-33
VX-16-661-115	3	homozygous for p.Phe508del or compound heterozygous for p.Phe508del and a resid-ual-function-mutation	6-11	8 weeks	Davies et al. J Cyst Fibros 2021; 20:68-77
K. Monotherapy with corrector GLPG222 or combination therapy with corrector GLPG2222 and potentiator ivacaftor					
NCT03119649 (FLAMINGO)	2	homozygous for p.Phe508del (monotherapy)	≥ 18	29 days	Bell et al. J Cyst Fibros 2019; 18:700-7
NCT03045523 (ALBATROSS)	2	heterozygous p.Phe508del/gating mutation	≥ 18	29 days	Bell et al. J Cyst Fibros 2019; 18:700-7

Study	Phase	*CFTR* mutation genotype	Age (yr)	Follow-up	Reference
L. Combination therapy of potentiator ABBV-3067 and corrector ABBV-2222					
AbbVie M19-530	2	homozygous for p.Phe508del	≥ 18	3 months	
M. Combination therapy with corrector GLPG2737, corrector lumacaftor and potentiator ivacaftor					
NCT03474042 (PELIKAN)	2	homozygous for p.Phe508del	≥ 18	28 days	van Koningsbruggen et al. J Cyst Fibros 2020;19:292-98
N. Combination therapy with corrector VX-152, corrector tezacaftor and potentiator ivacaftor					
VX-152-102	2	homozygous for p.Phe508del or compound heterozygous for p.Phe508del and a minimal function mutation	≥ 18	16 weeks	
O. Combination therapy with corrector VX-659, corrector tezacaftor and potentiator ivacaftor					
VX16-659-101; VX16-659-001	2	homozygous for p.Phe508del or compound heterozygous for p.Phe508del and a minimal function mutation	≥ 18	8 weeks	Davies et al. N Engl J Med 2018;379:1599-1611
VX17-659-102	3	heterozygous for p.Phe508del and a minimal function mutation	≥ 12	32 weeks	
VX17-659-103	3	homozygous for p.Phe508del	≥12	10 weeks	
P. Combination therapy with corrector elexacaftor, corrector tezacaftor and potentiator ivacaftor					
VX-445-101	2	homozygous for p.Phe508del or compound heterozygous for p.Phe508del and a minimal function mutation	≥ 18	12 weeks	Keating et al. N Engl J Med 2018;379:1612-1620
VX17-445-102	3	heterozygous for p.Phe508del and a minimal function mutation	≥ 12	24 weeks	Middleton et al. N Engl J Med 2019;381:1809-19
VX17-445-103	3	homozygous for p.Phe508del	≥ 12	8 weeks	Heijerman et al. Lancet 2019;394:1940-8
NCT03525574	3	Roll-over study of 002 and 003 participants	≥ 12	24 weeks	Griese et al. Am J Respir Crit Care Med 2021;203:381-5
NCT04378153 (SIMPLIFY)	4	Patients on ELE-TEZ-IVA treatment	≥ 12		Mayer-Hamblett et al. Ann Am Thorac Soc 2021;18: 1397-1405
VX18-445-104	3	p.Phe508del/gating or p.Phe508del/residual function genotypes	≥ 12	12 weeks	Barry et al. N Engl J Med 2021;385:815-25
VX18-445-106	3	homozygous for p.Phe508del or compound heterozygous for p.Phe508del and a minimal function mutation	6-11	32 weeks	Zemanick. Am J Respir Crit Care Med 2021;203:1522-32
VX18-445-109	3	homozygous for p.Phe508del	≥ 12	28 weeks	Sutharsan et al. Lancet Respir Med. 2021:S2213-2600(21) 00454-9
VX20-445-111 Part A	3	Patients with one or two p.Phe508 alleles	2-5	53 days	
VX20-445-116	3	heterozygous for p.Phe508del and a minimal function mutation	6-11	28 weeks	Mall, German CF Meeting 2021

Study	Phase	*CFTR* mutation genotype	Age (yr)	Follow-up	Reference
Q. Combination therapy with corrector posenacaftor (PTI-801), potentiator dirocaftor (PTI-808) and with or without amplifier PTI 428					
PTI-808-01	2	hetero- or homozygous for p.Phe508del	≥ 18	10 weeks	
R. Combination therapy of potentiator ABBV-2451 and corrector ABBV-2222 with or without corrector ABBV-2737					
NCT03540524 (FALCON)	1	hetero- or homozygous for p.Phe508del	≥ 18	28 days	
S. Combination therapy with corrector VX-121, corrector tezacaftor and potentiator VX-561					
VX18-121-101	2	homozygous for p.Phe508del or compound heterozygous for p.Phe508del and a minimal function mutation	≥ 18	17 weeks	
VX20-121-102	3	p.Phe508del/minimal function heterozygote	≥ 12	28 weeks	
VX20-121-103	3	homozygous for p.Phe508del or compound heterozygous for p.Phe508del and a gating or a residual function allele	≥ 12	28 weeks	
VX20-121-104	3	study participants of 121-102 or 121-103	≥ 12	96 weeks	
T. Inhalation therapy with CFTR mRNA MRT5005					
Translate Bio MRT5005-101	1/2	two class I or class II mutations	≥ 18	1 year	

Table 5.6: Clinical trials of CFTR correctors and CFTR potentiators in people with CF in the period 2007 – 2021.

conductance. Then the treatment with ivacaftor was investigated in patients with advanced lung disease (FEV1 < 40% pred; Hebestreit et al., 2013; Barry et al., 2014). Ivacaftor was found to be well tolerated and associated with weight gain and improved lung function. Whereas in patients with mild disease the increase in FEV1 was rapid and sustained, but showed a plateau effect by 3 months, the severely ill patients showed a slowly progressive increase in lung function without plateau.

The efficiency of ivacaftor in the early years of life is still the subject of clinical trials. Open-label studies demonstrated the efficacy and safety of ivacaftor in toddlers aged 12 to 24 months (Rosenfeld et al., 2018) and infants aged 4 to 12 months (Davies et al., 2021). Mean sweat chloride concentrations dropped by -73.5 (SD 17.5) mmol/L, which was more than 20 mmol/L higher than that recorded in adolescents and adults suggesting that CFTR modulation since the age at diagnosis more efficiently reverses the basic defect than a beginning later in life when irreversible organ damage had already been occurred. Consistent with this interpretation, the concentrations of fecal elastase-1 significantly increased within half a year of treatment with ivacaftor suggesting that exocrine pancreatic function is not irreversibly lost postpartum in CF but can be regained by restoration of CFTR function. Ongoing studies are now looking at the safety and effectiveness of ivacaftor during the first year of life. Thus, more than 15 years have meanwhile passed from the first administration of drug to a CF adult to the still ongoing tracking of ivacaftor's safety in CF neonates. Case reports and registries (Taylor-Cousar and Jain, 2021) are still the only source that documented the safety and efficacy of ivacaftor for fetus and pregnant women.

The administration of ivacaftor by CF patients with gating mutations is yet the only approved monotherapy with CFTR modulators. All other regimens consist of the combination of a CFTR potentiator with one or two CFTR correctors. The first approved indication has been the combination therapy with lumacaftor and ivacaftor for

Study	Drug(s)	Age (yr)	ppFEV1[a]	Weight (kg) *BMI (kg/m²)*	Pulmonary exacerba-tions	CFQ-R score[b]	Sweat chloride (mM)	$LCI_{2,5}$
Placebo-controlled studies								
VX08-770-102	ivacaftor	≥ 12	+10.6	+2.7	-55%	+8.6	-48	
VX08-770-103	ivacaftor	6-11	+12.5	+2.8		+7	-55	-2.2[c]
VX-770-110	ivacaftor	≥ 6	+2.1 (+5.0)[d]	ns	ns	+8.4	-24	
VX-770-111	ivacaftor	≥ 6	+10.7	*+0.7*		+8.9	-49	
VX-809-103/104	ivacaftor, lumacaftor	≥ 12	+2.9 – +3.3	*+0.24 – +0.28*	-30 – -39%	+2.2 – +3.1		
VX-809-109	ivacaftor, lumacaftor	6-11	+2.4				-21	-1.1
VX-661-106	tezacaftor, ivacaftor	≥ 12	+4.0	*+0.06*	-35%	+5.1	-10	
VX-661-107	tezacaftor, ivacaftor	≥ 12	+1.2 (ns)	*-0.02 (ns)*	-2% (ns)	+2.1 (ns)	-4	
VX-661-108	tezacaftor, ivacaftor	≥ 12	+6.8	*+0.16*	-46%	+11.1	-10	
VX-16-661-115	tezacaftor, ivacaftor	6-11	+2.8	+0.3		+2.3	-12	-0.5
VX17-445-102	elexa-, teza-, ivacaftor	≥ 12	+14.3	*+1.28*	-70%	+20.1	-49	
VX-445-116[e]	elexa-, teza-, ivacaftor	6-11	+11.0			+5.5	-51	-2.3
Active comparator-controlled studies								
VX-661-109	teza-, ivacaftor vs ivacaftor	≥ 12	+0.3			+2.8	-6	
VX17-445-103	elexa-, teza-, ivacaftor vs tezacaftor, ivacaftor	≥ 12	+12.8	*+1.18*	-70%	+13.8	-49	
VX18-445-104	elexa-, teza-, ivacaftor vs tezacaftor, ivacaftor	≥ 12	+3.5			+8.7	-23	
VX18-445-109	elexa-, teza-, ivacaftor vs tezacaftor, ivacaftor	≥ 12	+10.2			+15.9	-43	

Table 5.7: Outcome of phase 3, randomized, double-blind, controlled studies evaluating CFTR modulators in people with CF (FEV1 40-90% pred.). ns = no significant difference between treatment group and control group (placebo or active comparator), [a]percentage points FEV1 predicted, [b]points in the scheme of the 'Cystic Fibrosis Questionnaire – Revised (Respiratory domain)', [c]outcome of the clinical trial in patients with > 90% FEV1 and an increased 'lung clearance index' (LCI) higher than 7.4 (Davies et al. Lancet Respir Med 2013;1:630-8), [d]adults > 18 years, [e]no upper threshold for lung function (mean ppFEV1 at baseline: 89 percentage points; mean $LCI_{2,5}$ at baseline: 10.0).

p.Phe508del homozygotes. The large TRAFFIC and TRANSPORT trials with more than 1,000 study participants reported a modest improvement in FEV1 ranged from 2.6 to 4.0 absolute percentage points and a reduction of the rate of pulmonary exacerbations of 30-39% (☞ Table 5.7; Wainwright et al., 2015). Benefit continued with longer-term treatment. The subsequent roll-over study reported a mean gain in BMI of 0.96, a 35% reduction of pulmonary exacerbation rates and a 42% slower rate of $ppFEV_1$ decline than in matched registry controls at extension week 96 (Konstan et al., 2017; McColley et al., 2019). Thus, despite the substantially lower short-term benefit of LUM/IVA for p.Phe508del homozygotes than IVA for patients with gating mutations the combination therapy with LUM/IVA may pay off in the long run and therefore should be started early in life. Hence, the German Centre of Lung Research embarked on the worldwide first placebo-controlled, randomized, double-blind 96-week clinical trial in 2- to 5-year old preschoolers to test the efficacy of LUM/IVA to attenuate the progression of CF lung disease in clinically asymptomatic patients. The LCI derived from multiple-breath inert gas washout and the score evaluated from non-invasive magnetic resonance lung imaging were chosen as sensitive innovative endpoints. Small, but significant improvements in lung function and airway morphology were seen.

LUM/IVA was generally well tolerated, but a subgroup of patients complained during the initiation phase about dyspnea, wheezing, bronchial hyperreactivity or chest tightness, which was more frequently observed in patients with advanced lung disease. When patients with a FEV1 of < 40% were treated for the first time with LUM/IVA, they often experienced an acute decline in FEV1 that persisted for at least a day but resolved within the next 4 weeks (Popowicz et al., 2017). We therefore hospitalized all patients with advanced lung disease for the first three days of LUM/IVA therapy. Despite these precautions predominantly the elder patients often discontinued LUM/IVA therapy (Burgel et al., 2020). When this subgroup received tezacaftor instead of lumacaftor, combination therapy was not burdened anymore with respiratory adverse events (Schwarz et al., 2021).

Compared to LUM/IVA, the phase 3 trials with tezacaftor/ivacaftor in p.Phe508del homozygotes showed a slightly higher improvement of FEV1, a comparable reduction of the rate of pulmonary exacerbations, less respiratory adverse events and a lower gain of body weight (Taylor-Cousar et al., 2017; ☞ Table 5.7). The dual-combination regimen of TEZ/IVA did not have significantly greater clinical efficacy than IVA alone in patients with p.Phe508del/gating genotypes (McKone et al., 2021), but it substantively improved lung function and quality of life in compound heterozygotes for p.Phe508del and a residual function mutation who had been naïve for CFTR modulation (Rowe et al., 2017). Adolescents (12-18 years) and adults (> 18 years) increased their FEV1 by 12.0 and 6.0 absolute percentage points, respectively, which demonstrated a major difference in improvement between patients with still ongoing and completed body growth. During the 96-week open-label extension study the improvements of TEZ/IVA combination therapy were maintained (Flume et al., 2021). The annual rate of lung function decline was 61.5% (95% CI 35.8 to 86.1) lower in tezacaftor-ivacaftor-treated p.Phe508del/p.Phe508del participants than in matched registry controls; i.e. TEZ/IVA was 1.5-fold more efficacious than LUM/IVA in the reduction of FEV1 decline, the single most important predictor of survival in CF (Corey et al., 1997; Kim et al., 2018).

The next step in the evolution of clinical CFTR modulation turned out to be the major game changer: the introduction of triple therapy with elexacaftor/lumacaftor/ivacaftor. The phase 3 placebo-controlled and subsequent roll-over studies showed at week-24 sustained increases of 12 (CI 9.3 – 15.4) or even 15 (CI 12.9 – 16.3) absolute percentage points of FEV1 in p.Phe508del homozygotes and compound heterozygotes for p.Phe508 del and a minimal function mutation compared to placebo, respectively (Heijerman et al., 2019; Middleton et al., 2019; Sutharsan et al., 2021; ☞ Table 5.7). Correspondingly, the study participants scored their improvements in quality of life by 14 and 20 points, which was qualified by study participants as 'never expected', 'fantastic' or 'incredible'. For comparison, a gain of only 4 points is already qualified as clinically relevant. By week-48, the rate of pulmonary exacerbations had decreased by 70%. Sweat chloride concentrations were in the pathological range at baseline, but during exposure to ELX/TEZ/IVA dropped by a mean 50 mmol/L into the intermediary or even normal range in the majority of patients implying that the basic defect of defective chloride reabsorption in the sweat duct had been partially or completely reversed by triple therapy.

Subsequent comparator studies demonstrated that ELX/TEZ/IVA further enhanced lung function, anthropometry and quality of life of patients with gating and residual function mutations who already administered efficient CFTR modulator therapy with ivacaftor and tezacaftor/ivacaftor, respectively (Barry et al., 2021). So, what's next? There remains the holy grail to develop even more effective CFTR modulators that can restore CFTR function toward levels seen in carriers (who do not develop CF) in as many patients with CF as possible. This ambitious goal will be pursued in the upcoming 48-week phase 3 studies that will benchmark the triple therapy with the novel corrector VX-121, tezacaftor and deuterated ivacaftor against ELX/TEZ/IVA in patients who are homozygous for p.Phe508del or who are compound heterozygous for a gating, a residual function or a minimal function mutation (EudraCT Numbers: 2021-000694-85; 2021-000712-31).

The CFTR modulators that were tested in phase 3 trials, are meanwhile available to all age groups whereby the European Medical Agency (EMA) is still somewhat more restrictive in its label than the FDA.

The monotherapy with ivacaftor (trade name Kalydeco®) can be prescribed in the US for patients of 4 months or older carrying at least one of 33 mutations the majority of which are gating mutations including p.Gly551Asp and p.Arg117His as the most frequent mutations. In patients age 2 years and older ivacaftor is indicated for the treatment of CF who have one mutation in the *CFTR* gene that is responsive to ivacaftor based on clinical and/or *in vitro* assay data (FDA, September 2020).

Lumacaftor/ivacaftor (trade name Orkambi®) is indicated for patients age 2 years and older who are homozygous for p.Phe508del (FDA, August 2018).

Tezacaftor/ivacaftor (trade names Symdeko®/ Symkevi®) is indicated for the treatment of CF patients age 6 years and older who are homozygous for p.Phe508del or who carry at least one mutation in the *CFTR* gene that is responsive to tezacaftor/ivacaftor based on *in vitro* data and/or clinical evidence (FDA, December 2020).

Elexacaftor/tezacaftor/ivacaftor (trade names Trikafta® in North America and Australia, Kaftrio® in Europe) is indicated for the treatment of CF patients age 6 years and older who carry at least one p.Phe508del allele or at least one specified mutation known to respond to Trikafta *in vitro* (FDA, June 2021). The current label lists 148 mutations consisting of 4 in-frame deletions /insertions including p.Phe508del and 144 missense mutations.

Special restrictions apply to co-morbidities like liver disease or co-medications causing clinically significant drug-drug interactions (☞ Chapter 5.2.).

The list of approved mutations surprisingly includes sequence variants

- a) known to be associated with CFTR-RD (p.Arg 75Gln, p.Arg117Cys, p.Lys206Trp, p.Leu997 Phe, p.Asp1152His),
- b) that are lowly responsive to CFTR modulation based on *in vitro* assay data (p.Arg347Pro),
- c) that yielded discrepant results in assays *in vitro* and *in vivo* (p.Glu92Lys, p.Met1101Lys),
- d) that were validated to confer normal CFTR function in ICM and NPD (p.Val201Met),
- e) that were classified by the CF Genetic Analysis Consortium as polymorphisms (p.Phe508Cys, p.Arg668Cys).

The presence of mutations of category a, d and e as a disease-causing lesion in a CF patient is unlikely.

5.4. Post-approval studies

Burkhard Tümmler

Almost all phase 3 trials examined the clinical response to modulators in cohorts with moderate lung disease as indicated by a spirometry of ppFEV1 of 40 -90%. Considering their bleak prognosis, patients with a more impaired lung function are in most urgent need to have access to CFTR modulators. Hence, prior to the official approval by the regulatory authorities 'compassionate use' programs have been regularly launched for this vulnerable patient group (Hebestreit et al., 2013; Wood et al., 2013; Salvatore et al., 2020). These patients were at a higher risk that they could not cope with the drainage of massive mucus plugs that were immediately mobilized after the initiation of modulator therapy. Typical adverse events were severe headache caused by mobilized secretions in the sinuses, upper abdominal pain when mobilized gallstones passed the bile duct and shortness of breath when mobilized mucus plugs were drained into the larger conducting airways. The latter complication could be severe or even life–threatening if an individual with end stage lung disease was physically not capable anymore to actively expectorate large amounts of sputum (Burgel et al., 2020; 2021). Conversely, the impact of treatment was often encouraging for dual combination therapy and even spectacular with the novel triple therapy. For example, lumacaftor/ivacaftor or tezacaftor/ivacaftor reduced lung function decline and the rate of pulmonary exacerbations and improved lung function, physical performance and quality of life (Wark et al., 2019; Ejiofor et al., 2020; Tong et al., 2020; Schwarz et al., 2021). Even more striking, many patients waiting for a lung transplant were removed from the list within a few weeks of treatment with ELX/TEZ/IVA, gained weight and improved FEV1 by a mean 15 percentage points (Burgel et al., 2021; Stylemans et al., 2021).

With the exception of the early days of the clinical development of ivacaftor and lumacaftor (Accurso et al., 2010; Clancy et al., 2012), the sweat chloride concentration has been applied as the only CFTR biomarker to demonstrate the ability of a drug to influence the basic defect. Hence, other CFTR biomarkers have been examined later in post-approval studies.

ICM and NPD

Under ivacaftor or dual lumacaftor/ivacaftor therapy the chloride secretory responses of the intestinal epithelium increased to 50-60% of normal in CF patients with gating mutations (Graeber et al., 2015) and to about 20% of normal in p.Phe508del homozygous patients, respectively (Graeber et al., 2018; Masson et al., 2020). More efficiently, exposure to ELX/TEZ/IVA shifted mutant CFTR-mediated chloride secretory activity into the normal range of the ICM for most patients who carry at least one p.Phe508del allele (Graeber et al., 2022). CFTR-mediated chloride conductance of the upper respiratory epithelium improved to a mean 18-20% of normal with LUM/IVA (Graeber et al., 2018; Masson et al., 2020) and to a mean 47% of normal with ELX/LUM/IVA (Graeber et al., 2022). CFTR apical expression was increased by lumacaftor or tezacaftor to about 22% of wild-type level in p.Phe508del homozygous nasal epithelial cells (Pranke et al., 2017). Thus, treatment with ELX/ TEZ/IVA results in effective improvement of CFTR function in airway and intestinal epithelia in patients with CF and one or two p.Phe508 alleles.

Sweat test and sweat secretion tests

Treatment with IVA in patients with at least one p.Gly551Asp allele or treatment with ELX/LUM/IVA in patients with at least one p.Phe508del allele commonly normalized the chloride reabsorption in the sweat duct. Conversely, the β-adrenergic stimulated sweat secretion in the coil reached just about 5% of median wild type β-adrenergic sweat rate (Accurso et al., 2014; Char et al., 2014; 2017; Kim et al., 2018; Pallenberg et al., 2021). Apparently β-adrenergic sweat stimulation in the coil is more stringent in its requirements for a wild type CFTR conformation whereas the reabsorption of chloride in the sweat duct tolerates residual structural and functional deficits of pharmacologically rescued mutant CFTR in the apical membrane. The limited response of the β-adrenergic sweat rate to high-efficient CFTR modulation allows the evaluation of new, potentially even more efficient CFTR modulators in the future, while the sweat chloride concentration may already have reached the limit of its sensitivity.

The effect of the exposure of CFTR modulators to non-epithelial host defense cells is of general relevance for the understanding of the molecular pathology of CF because the data in the literature are contradictory. Targeting CFTR in monocytes and thereof derived macrophages provided conflicting evidence of whether CFTR regulates phagosome acidification in macrophages and therefore alters bactericidal activity (Di et al., 2006; Haggie and Verkman, 2007). Numerous reports have meanwhile demonstrated that treatment with CFTR modulators improves the function of CF defense cells implying that CFTR is indeed critically involved in non-epithelial host defense. Ivacaftor increased chloride efflux, reduced the responsiveness to interferon γ in monocytes (Guerra et al., 2017; Hisert et al., 2020) and modulated the expression of genes related to cell differentiation, microbial infection, inflammation, Toll-like receptor signaling, and metabolism (Sun et al., 2019). The pool of circulating neutrophils was less activated but retained the potential to migrate and phagocytose when needed (Hardisty et al., 2021). Lumacaftor alone restored the ability of CF monocyte-derived macrophages to phagocytose and kill *P. aeruginosa* to non-CF wild-type levels (Barnaby et al., 2018). Different CFTR modulator combinations downregulate inflammation differently in CF (Jarosz-Griffiths et al., 2020). Exposure of activated CF monocytes to lumacaftor/ivacaftor or tezacaftor/ivacaftor consistently decreased the levels of IL-18, whereas IL-1β was only reduced with ivacaftor/tezacaftor. In summary, host defense cells are a target of CFTR modulators.

Besides these studies of the impact of CFTR modulators on the intracellular and secretory functions of CFTR, multi-center longitudinal cohort studies determined the response of clinically relevant markers in the post-approval setting (reviews: Sergeev et al., 2020; Duckers et al., 2021). For example, CFTR modulators, alone or in combination, substantially reduced the risk of recurrent acute pancreatitis over a mean follow-up period of 3 years in adult patients with PS-CF and a history of prior acute pancreatitis (Akshintala et al., 2019).

Most studies dealt with ivacaftor, the first drug that made it to the clinic. Ivacaftor attenuated inflammation and clinical symptoms of sinonasal and lung disease, reduced extra-oesophageal reflux, restored bile acid homeostasis and improved nutritional status, bone microarchitecture, mucociliary clearance, smooth muscle tone, airway surface liquid and intestinal pH profile, but did not attenuate CF-related diabetes and failed to activate β-adrenergic sweat secretion (Rowe et al., 2014; Heltshe et al., 2015; Bernarde et al., 2015; Sheikh et al., 2015; Adam et al., 2016; Borowitz et al., 2016; Gelfond et al., 2017; Hisert et al., 2017; Zeybel et al., 2017; Abou Alaiwa et al., 2018; van de Peppel et al., 2019; Einarsson et al., 2021; Mainz et al., 2021; Putman et al., 2021). Exocrine pancreatic function improved in preschoolers (Nichols et al., 2020). One- to 12-month ivacaftor treatment did not modulate the airway microbiome (Peleg et al., 2018; Harris et al., 2020; Kristensen et al., 2021), but long-term treatment reduced the prevalence of typical pathogens such as *S. aureus, P. aeruginosa* and *Aspergillus* spp. (Frost et al., 2019). The rate of annual pulmonary exacerbations was reduced by 50% irrespective of an acute response to IVA within the first months of treatment implying that the absence of an acute response does not rule out long-term benefit (Sawicki et al., 2015; Heltshe et al., 2018). Unexpectedly, ivacaftor-treated females with CF had a greater reduction in pulmonary exacerbations than males with CF (Secunda et al., 2020). The improvements in growth, quality of life measures, sweat chloride, *P. aeruginosa* detection, and pulmonary exacerbation rates requiring antimicrobial therapy persisted through three to thirteen years of therapy demonstrating the long-term benefits and disease modifying effects of ivacaftor (Sawicki et al., 2015; Hubert et al., 2018; Higgins et al., 2020; Guimbellot et al., 2021; Hubert et al., 2021; Kawala et al., 2021; Thorat et al., 2021). Data from the US and UK CF patient registries from the years 2011-2016 showed that in a real-world setting relative to comparators, ivacaftor-treated patients had better preserved lung function (mean change in percent predicted FEV_1, -0.7 percentage points with ivacaftor vs -8.3 percentage points in comparators) and improved nutritional status (mean body mass index change +2.4 kg/m^2 with ivacaftor vs +1.6 kg/m^2 in comparators; Volkova et al., 2020). However, if a pulmonary exacerbation happens, ivacaftor does not influence the outcome suggesting that the recovery of lung function is not affected by CFTR modulation (Flume et al., 2018). Voluntary or accidental withdrawal of treatment with ivacaftor is risky. Cessation of treatment can lead to dramatic rapid decline of patient's lung function and symptoms (Trimble and Donaldson, 2018).

Lumacaftor/ivacaftor in p.Phe508del homozygotes turned out to be less efficacious than ivacaftor in patients with gating mutations. The outcome of the post-approval studies was not consistent. In an observational study performed at four study sites in the US, sweat chloride improved by 18 mmol/L, indicating a modest restoration of CFTR activity, but no demonstrable change in FEV1, lung clearance index, mucociliary clearance or insulin secretion were observed (Donaldson et al., 2021; Moheet et al., 2021). In the French and Greek patient populations, LUM/IVA led to a modest 3% or 4.3% increase in ppFEV1 in patients with intermediary lung disease with LCI being stable, but did not change lung function in patients with normal (> 90%) or strongly compromised (< 40%) spirometry (Burgel et al., 2021a; Loukou et al., 2020; Reix et al., 2021). The US PROSPECT consortium saw no significant changes in lung function as measured by spirometry with clinical initiation of LUM/IVA, but detected a favorable decrease of the LCI of 0.6-0.8 units within one year of follow-up (Shaw et al., 2020). However, LUM/IVA reduced peribronchial thickening and airway mucous plugging (Arnaud et al., 2021), delayed the acquisition of CF pathogens (Singh et al., 2019) and reduced bacterial load with *P. aeruginosa* within the lung (Neerincx et al., 2021). Since long-term survival benefits of LUM/IVA cannot yet be quantified, Rubin et al. (2019) performed a simulation study based on existing registry and clinical trial data. Initiating LUM/IVA at ages 6, 12, 18, and 25 years and assuming lifetime treatment resulted in incremental median predicted survival of 23.4, 18.2, 11.0, and 4.8 years, respectively. The authors assumed that the standard care is retained, but in the real-world treatment patterns will change over time (☞ below).

Post-approval multi-center studies on ELX/TEZ/IVA have just been started (Nichols et al., 2021a). The first post-approval study on a large cohort of 487 people with CF reported on an improvement of FEV_1 of 9.8 absolute percentage points after 6 months of ELX/TEZ/IVA therapy (Nichols et al., 2021b). Moreover, reversion of some 'irreversible' symptoms of CF disease have already been described: ELX/TEZ/IVA reduced sinus opacification (Beswick et al., 2021) and resolved subfertility in females (O'Connor et al., 2021). Fortner et al. (2021) reported on the first healthy newborn with two CF-causing *CFTR* mutations born to a p.Phe508del homozygous mother taking ELX/TEZ/IVA throughput pregnancy. Conversely, a few severe adverse events have also been reported: ELX/TEZ/IVA caused mental health problems (Heo et al., 2021), acute liver injury (Lowry et al., 2021) or mobilization of gallstones and subsequent cholecystitis in a few patients (Safirstein et al., 2021).

Adherence is an important goal for CF management, as non-adherence is linked to poor health outcomes. Annual medication adherence to IVA, LUM/IVA and TEZ/IVA of the UK patient population has been extracted from data of the national specialty pharmacy database (Mehta et al., 2021). The mean proportion of days covered by medication was 0.80. Adherence to medication was higher in children than in adults. Clinical efficacy of treatment is high, and the medication is extremely expensive. Thus, the authors concluded that the rates of adherence need to be improved in people with CF.

Ivacaftor became available to people with CF about ten years ago. Hence, long-term changes in treatment patterns can now be extracted from registry data. In the UK a clear divergence in treatment use over time was seen between individuals treated with ivacaftor and those untreated due to their genotype for a number of long-term treatments widely used in CF, including dornase alfa, hypertonic saline and inhaled antibiotics (Granger et al., 2021). Differences in treatment use were most pronounced for children and for those with high lung function. Treatment burden in CF is high and ways to simplify this burden have been recognised as a priority area for clinical trials. Current or planned randomised controlled trials SIMPLIFY (Clinical Trials.gov: NCT04378153) and CF STORM (EudraCT number 2020-005864-77) aim to assess treatment simplification for mucoactive nebulised therapies in patients on elexacaftor-tezacaftor-ivacaftor. Understanding the association between change in treatment patterns and clinical outcomes is important to help interpret real-world effectiveness data and to help patients' and clinical care team's decision making, particularly if there is any deviation from an anticipated degree of efficacy that may have been expected from the original phase III clinical trials (Granger et al., 2021).

5.5. References

Abou Alaiwa MH, Launspach JL, Grogan B, Carter S, Zabner J, Stoltz DA, Singh PK, McKone EF, Welsh MJ. Ivacaftor-induced sweat chloride reductions correlate with increases in airway surface liquid pH in cystic fibrosis. JCI Insight 2018;3:e121468. doi: 10.1172/jci.insight.121468.

Accurso FJ, Rowe SM, Clancy JP, Boyle MP, Dunitz JM, Durie PR, Sagel SD, Hornick DB, Konstan MW, Donaldson SH, Moss RB, Pilewski JM, Rubenstein RC, Uluer AZ, Aitken ML, Freedman SD, Rose LM, Mayer-Hamblett N, Dong Q, Zha J, Stone AJ, Olson ER, Ordoñez CL, Campbell PW, Ashlock MA, Ramsey BW. Effect of VX-770 in persons with cystic fibrosis and the G551D-CFTR mutation. N Engl J Med 2010;363:1991-2003. doi: 10.1056/NEJMoa0909825.

Accurso FJ, Van Goor F, Zha J, Stone AJ, Dong Q, Ordonez CL, Rowe SM, Clancy JP, Konstan MW, Hoch HE, Heltshe SL, Ramsey BW, Campbell PW, Ashlock MA. Sweat chloride as a biomarker of CFTR activity: proof of concept and ivacaftor clinical trial data. J Cyst Fibros 2014;13:139-47. doi: 10.1016/j.jcf.2013.09.007.

Adam RJ, Hisert KB, Dodd JD, Grogan B, Launspach JL, Barnes JK, Gallagher CG, Sieren JP, Gross TJ, Fischer AJ, Cavanaugh JE, Hoffman EA, Singh PK, Welsh MJ, Mc Kone EF, Stoltz DA. Acute administration of ivacaftor to people with cystic fibrosis and a G551D-CFTR mutation reveals smooth muscle abnormalities. JCI Insight 2016; 1:e86183. doi: 10.1172/jci.insight.86183.

Akshintala VS, Kamal A, Faghih M, Cutting GR, Cebotaru L, West NE, Jennings MT, Dezube R, Whitcomb DC, Lechtzin N, Merlo CA, Singh VK. Cystic fibrosis transmembrane conductance regulator modulators reduce the risk of recurrent acute pancreatitis among adult patients with pancreas sufficient cystic fibrosis. Pancreatology 2019;19:1023-1026. doi: 10.1016/j.pan.2019.09.014.

Anderson JD, Liu Z, Odom LV, Kersh L, Guimbellot JS. CFTR function and clinical response to modulators parallel nasal epithelial organoid swelling. Am J Physiol Lung Cell Mol Physiol 2021;321:L119-L129. doi: 10.1152/ajplung.00639.2020.

Arnaud F, Stremler-Le Bel N, Reynaud-Gaubert M, Mancini J, Gaubert JY, Gorincour G. Computed tomographic changes in patients with cystic fibrosis treated by combination therapy with lumacaftor and ivacaftor. J Clin Med 2021;10:1999. doi: 10.3390/jcm10091999.

Barnaby R, Koeppen K, Nymon A, Hampton TH, Berwin B, Ashare A, Stanton BA. Lumacaftor (VX-809) restores the ability of CF macrophages to phagocytose and kill Pseudomonas aeruginosa. Am J Physiol Lung Cell Mol Physiol 2018;314:L432-L438. doi: 10.1152/ajplung.00461.2017.

Barry PJ, Plant BJ, Nair A, Bicknell S, Simmonds NJ, Bell NJ, Shafi NT, Daniels T, Shelmerdine S, Felton I, Gunaratnam C, Jones AM, Horsley AR. Effects of ivacaftor in patients with cystic fibrosis who carry the G551D mutation and have severe lung disease. Chest. 2014;146: 152-158. doi: 10.1378/chest.13-2397.

Barry PJ, Mall MA, Álvarez A, Colombo C, de Winter-de Groot KM, Fajac I, McBennett KA, McKone EF, Ramsey BW, Sutharsan S, Taylor-Cousar JL, Tullis E, Ahluwalia N, Jun LS, Moskowitz SM, Prieto-Centurion V, Tian S, Waltz D, Xuan F, Zhang Y, Rowe SM, Polineni D; VX18-445-104 Study Group. Triple therapy for cystic fibrosis Phe508del-gating and -residual function genotypes. N Engl J Med 2021;385:815-825. doi: 10.1056/NEJMoa2100665.

Becq F, Mirval S, Carrez T, Lévêque M, Billet A, Coraux C, Sage E, Cantereau A. The rescue of F508del-CFTR by elexacaftor/tezacaftor/ivacaftor (Trikafta) in human airway epithelial cells is underestimated due to the presence of ivacaftor. Eur Respir J 2021:2100671. doi: 10.1183/13993003.00671-2021.

Bell SC, Barry PJ, De Boeck K, Drevinek P, Elborn JS, Plant BJ, Miniæ P, Van Braeckel E, Verhulst S, Muller K, Kanters D, Bellaire S, de Kock H, Geller DE, Conrath K, Van de Steen O, van der Ent K. CFTR activity is enhanced by the novel corrector GLPG2222, given with and without ivacaftor in two randomized trials. J Cyst Fibros 2019;18:700-7. doi: 10.1016/j.jcf.2019.04.014

Bengtson CD, He J, Kim MD, Salathe MA. Cystic fibrosis-related diabetes is associated with worse lung function trajectory despite ivacaftor use. Am J Respir Crit Care Med 2021;204:1343-1345. doi: 10.1164/rccm.202104-1060 LE.

Bernarde C, Keravec M, Mounier J, Gouriou S, Rault G, Férec C, Barbier G, Héry-Arnaud G. Impact of the CFTR-potentiator ivacaftor on airway microbiota in cystic fibrosis patients carrying a G551D mutation. PLoS One 2015;10:e0124124. doi: 10.1371/journal.pone.0124124.

Beswick DM, Humphries SM, Balkissoon CD, Strand M, Vladar EK, Lynch DA, Taylor-Cousar JL. Impact of CFTR therapy on chronic rhinosinusitis and health status: Deep learning CT analysis and patient reported outcomes. Ann Am Thorac Soc 2022;19:12-19. doi: 10.1513/AnnalsATS.202101-057OC.

Boinot C, Jollivet Souchet M, Ferru-Clément R, Becq F. Searching for combinations of small-molecule correctors to restore F508del-cystic fibrosis transmembrane conductance regulator function and processing. J Pharmacol Exp Ther 2014;350:624-34. doi: 10.1124/jpet.114.214890.

Borowitz D, Lubarsky B, Wilschanski M, Munck A, Gelfond D, Bodewes F, Schwarzenberg SJ. Nutritional status improved in cystic fibrosis patients with the G551D mutation after treatment with ivacaftor. Dig Dis Sci. 2016; 61:198-207. doi: 10.1007/s10620-015-3834-2.

Boyle MP, Bell SC, Konstan MW, McColley SA, Rowe SM, Rietschel E, Huang X, Waltz D, Patel NR, Rodman D; VX09-809-102 study group. A CFTR corrector (lumacaftor) and a CFTR potentiator (ivacaftor) for treatment of patients with cystic fibrosis who have a phe508del CFTR mutation: a phase 2 randomised controlled trial. Lancet Respir Med 2014;2:527-38. doi: 10.1016/S2213-2600(14)70132-8.

Brindani N, Gianotti A, Giovani S, Giacomina F, Di Fruscia P, Sorana F, Bertozzi SM, Ottonello G, Goldoni L, Penna I, Russo D, Summa M, Bertorelli R, Ferrera L, Pesce E, Sondo E, Galietta LJV, Bandiera T, Pedemonte N, Bertozzi F. Identification, structure-activity relationship, and biological characterization of 2,3,4,5-Tetrahydro-1-H-pyrido[4,3-b]indoles as a novel class of CFTR potentiators. J Med Chem 2020;63:11169-94. doi: 10.1021/acs.jmedchem.0c01050.

Burgel PR, Durieu I, Chiron R, Mely L, Prevotat A, Murris-Espin M, Porzio M, Abely M, Reix P, Marguet C, Macey J, Sermet-Gaudelus I, Corvol H, Bui S, Biouhee T, Hubert D, Munck A, Lemonnier L, Dehillotte C, Silva JD, Paillasseur JL, Martin C; French Cystic Fibrosis Reference Network study group. Clinical response to lumacaftor-ivacaftor in patients with cystic fibrosis according to baseline lung function. J Cyst Fibros. 2021;20:220-227. doi: 10.1016/j.jcf.2020.06.012.

Burgel PR, Munck A, Durieu I, Chiron R, Mely L, Prevotat A, Murris-Espin M, Porzio M, Abely M, Reix P, Marguet C, Macey J, Sermet-Gaudelus I, Corvol H, Bui S, Lemonnier L, Dehillotte C, Da Silva J, Paillasseur JL, Hubert D; French Cystic Fibrosis Reference Network Study Group. Real-life safety and effectiveness of Lumacaftor-Ivacaftor in patients with cystic fibrosis. Am J Respir Crit Care Med 2020; 201:188-197. doi: 10.1164/rccm.201906-1227OC.

Burgel PR, Durieu I, Chiron R, Ramel S, Danner-Boucher I, Prevotat A, Grenet D, Marguet C, Reynaud-Gaubert M, Macey J, Mely L, Fanton A, Quetant S, Lemonnier L, Paillasseur JL, Da Silva J, Martin C; French Cystic Fibrosis Reference Network Study Group. Rapid improvement after starting Elexacaftor-Tezacaftor-Ivacaftor in patients with cystic fibrosis and advanced pulmonary disease. Am J Respir Crit Care Med 2021;204:64-73. doi: 10.1164/rccm.202011-4153OC.

Byrnes LJ, Xu Y, Qiu X, Hall JD, West GM. Sites associated with Kalydeco binding on human Cystic Fibrosis Transmembrane Conductance Regulator revealed by hydrogen/deuterium exchange. Sci Rep. 2018;8:4664. doi: 10.1038/s41598-018-22959-6.

Capurro V, Tomati V, Sondo E, Renda M, Borrelli A, Pastorino C, Guidone D, Venturini A, Giraudo A, Mandrup Bertozzi S, Musante I, Bertozzi F, Bandiera T, Zara F, Galietta LJV, Pedemonte N. Partial rescue of F508del-CFTR stability and trafficking defects by double corrector treatment. Int J Mol Sci 2021;22:5262. doi: 10.3390/ijms22105262.

Char JE, Dunn C, Davies Z, Milla C, Moss RB, Wine JJ. The magnitude of ivacaftor effects on fluid secretion via R117H-CFTR channels: Human in vivo measurements. PLoS One 2017;12:e0175486. doi: 10.1371/journal.pone.0175486.

Char JE, Wolfe MH, Cho HJ, Park IH, Jeong JH, Frisbee E, Dunn C, Davies Z, Milla C, Moss RB, Thomas EA, Wine JJ. A little CFTR goes a long way: CFTR-dependent sweat secretion from G551D and R117H-5T cystic fibrosis subjects taking ivacaftor. PLoS One. 2014;9:e88564. doi: 10.1371/journal.pone.0088564.

Chilvers MA, Davies JC, Milla C, Tian S, Han Z, Cornell AG, Owen CA, Ratjen F. Long-term safety and efficacy of lumacaftor-ivacaftor therapy in children aged 6-11 years with cystic fibrosis homozygous for the F508del-CFTR mutation: a phase 3, open-label, extension study. Lancet Respir Med 2021;9:721-732. doi: 10.1016/S2213-2600(20)30517-8.

Chin S, Hung M, Won A, Wu YS, Ahmadi S, Yang D, Elmallah S, Toutah K, Hamilton CM, Young RN, Viirre RD, Yip CM, Bear CE. Lipophilicity of the cystic fibrosis drug, Ivacaftor (VX-770), and its destabilizing effect on the major CF-causing mutation: F508del. Mol Pharmacol 2018;94:917-25. doi: 10.1124/mol.118.112177.

Cholon DM, Quinney NL, Fulcher ML, Esther CR Jr, Das J, Dokholyan NV, Randell SH, Boucher RC, Gentzsch M. Potentiator ivacaftor abrogates pharmacological correction of ΔF508 CFTR in cystic fibrosis. Sci Transl Med 2014;6:246ra96. doi: 10.1126/scitranslmed.3008680.

Clancy JP, Rowe SM, Accurso FJ, Aitken ML, Amin RS, Ashlock MA, Ballmann M, Boyle MP, Bronsveld I, Campbell PW, De Boeck K, Donaldson SH, Dorkin HL, Dunitz JM, Durie PR, Jain M, Leonard A, McCoy KS, Moss RB, Pilewski JM, Rosenbluth DB, Rubenstein RC, Schechter MS, Botfield M, Ordoñez CL, Spencer-Green GT, Vernillet L, Wisseh S, Yen K, Konstan MW. Results of a phase IIa study of VX-809, an investigational CFTR corrector compound, in subjects with cystic fibrosis homozygous for the F508del-CFTR mutation. Thorax 2012;67:12-8. doi: 10.1136/thoraxjnl-2011-200393.

Corey M, Edwards L, Levison H, Knowles M. Longitudinal analysis of pulmonary function decline in patients with cystic fibrosis. J Pediatr. 1997;131:809-14. doi: 10.1016/s0022-3476(97)70025-8

Csanády L, Töröcsik B. Cystic fibrosis drug ivacaftor stimulates CFTR channels at picomolar concentrations. Elife 2019;8:e46450. doi: 10.7554/eLife.46450.

Davies G, Rowbotham NJ, Smith S, Elliot ZC, Gathercole K, Rayner O, Leighton PA, Herbert S, Duff AJ, Chandran S, Daniels T, Nash EF, Smyth AR. Characterising burden of treatment in cystic fibrosis to identify priority areas for clinical trials. J Cyst Fibros. 2020;19:499-502. doi: 10.1016/j.jcf.2019.10.025.

Davies JC, Cunningham S, Harris WT, Lapey A, Regelmann WE, Sawicki GS, Southern KW, Robertson S, Green Y, Cooke J, Rosenfeld M; KIWI Study Group. Safety, pharmacokinetics, and pharmacodynamics of ivacaftor in patients aged 2-5 years with cystic fibrosis and a CFTR gating mutation (KIWI): an open-label, single-arm study. Lancet Respir Med 2016;4:107-15. doi: 10.1016/S2213-2600(15)00545-7.

Davies JC, Moskowitz SM, Brown C, Horsley A, Mall MA, McKone EF, Plant BJ, Prais D, Ramsey BW, Taylor-Cousar JL, Tullis E, Uluer A, McKee CM, Robertson S, Shilling RA, Simard C, Van Goor F, Waltz D, Xuan F, Young T, Rowe SM; VX16-659-101 Study Group. VX-659-Tezacaftor-Ivacaftor in patients with cystic fibrosis and one or two Phe508del alleles. N Engl J Med 2018;379:1599-1611. doi: 10.1056/NEJMoa1807119

Davies JC, Sermet-Gaudelus I, Naehrlich L, Harris RS, Campbell D, Ahluwalia N, Short C, Haseltine E, Panorchan P, Saunders C, Owen CA, Wainwright CE; VX16-661-115 Investigator Group. A phase 3, double-blind, parallel-group study to evaluate the efficacy and safety of tezacaftor in combination with ivacaftor in participants 6 through 11 years of age with cystic fibrosis homozygous for F508del or heterozygous for the F508del-CFTR mutation and a residual function mutation. J Cyst Fibros 2021; 20:68-77. doi: 10.1016/j.jcf.2020.07.023.

Davies J, Sheridan H, Bell N, Cunningham S, Davis SD, Elborn JS, Milla CE,Starner TD, Weiner DJ, Lee PS, Ratjen F. Assessment of clinical response to ivacaftor with lung clearance index in cystic fibrosis patients with a G551D-CFTR mutation and preserved spirometry: a randomised controlled trial. Lancet Respir Med 2013; 1:630-8. doi: 10.1016/S2213-2600(13)70182-6.

Davies JC, Van de Steen O, van Koningsbruggen-Rietschel S, Drevinek P, Derichs N, McKone EF, Kanters D, Allamassey L, Namour F, de Kock H, Conrath K. GLPG1837, a CFTR potentiator, in p.Gly551Asp (G551D)-CF patients: An open-label, single-arm, phase 2a study (SAPHIRA1). J Cyst Fibros 2019;18:693-9. doi: 10.1016/j.jcf.2019.05.006.

Davies JC, Wainwright CE, Canny GJ, Chilvers MA, Howenstine MS, Munck A, Mainz JG, Rodriguez S, Li H, Yen K, Ordoñez CL, Ahrens R; VX08-770-103 (ENVISION) Study Group. Efficacy and safety of ivacaftor in patients aged 6 to 11 years with cystic fibrosis with a G551D mutation. Am J Respir Crit Care Med 2013;187: 1219-25. doi: 10.1164/rccm.201301-0153OC.

Davies JC, Wainwright CE, Sawicki GS, Higgins MN, Campbell D, Harris C, Panorchan P, Haseltine E, Tian S, Rosenfeld M. Ivacaftor in infants aged 4 to <12 months with cystic fibrosis and a gating mutation. Results of a two-part phase 3 clinical trial. Am J Respir Crit Care Med 2021;203:585-93. doi: 10.1164/rccm.202008-3177OC.

De Boeck K, Munck A, Walker S, Faro A, Hiatt P, Gilmartin G, Higgins M. Efficacy and safety of ivacaftor in patients with cystic fibrosis and a non-G551D gating mutation. J Cyst Fibros 2014;13:674-80. doi: 10.1016/j.jcf.2014.09.005.

de Poel E, Spelier S, Korporaal R, Lai KW, Boj SF, Conrath K, van der Ent CK, Beekman JM. CFTR Rescue in intestinal organoids with GLPG/ABBV-2737, ABBV/GLPG-2222 and ABBV/GLPG-2451 triple therapy. Front Mol Biosci. 2021;8:698358. doi: 10.3389/fmolb.2021.698358.

Dekkers JF, Wiegerinck CL, de Jonge HR, Bronsveld I, Janssens HM, de Winter-de Groot KM, Brandsma AM, de Jong NW, Bijvelds MJ, Scholte BJ, Nieuwenhuis EE, van den Brink S, Clevers H, van der Ent CK, Middendorp S, Beekman JM. A functional CFTR assay using primary cystic fibrosis intestinal organoids. Nat Med. 2013;19: 939-45. doi: 10.1038/nm.3201.

Dekkers JF, Gogorza Gondra RA, Kruisselbrink E, Vonk AM, Janssens HM, de Winter-de Groot KM, van der Ent CK, Beekman JM. Optimal correction of distinct CFTR folding mutants in rectal cystic fibrosis organoids. Eur Respir J. 2016;48:451-8. doi: 10.1183/13993003.01192-2015.

Dekkers JF, Berkers G, Kruisselbrink E, Vonk A, de Jonge HR, Janssens HM, Bronsveld I, van de Graaf EA, Nieuwenhuis EE, Houwen RH, Vleggaar FP, Escher JC, de Rijke YB, Majoor CJ, Heijerman HG, de Winter-de Groot KM, Clevers H, van der Ent CK, Beekman JM. Characterizing responses to CFTR-modulating drugs using rectal organoids derived from subjects with cystic fibrosis. Sci Transl Med. 2016;8:344ra84. doi: 10.1126/scitranslmed.aad8278.

Derichs N, Taylor-Cousar JL, Davies JC, Fajac I, Tullis E, Nazareth D, Downey DG, Rosenbluth D, Malfroot A, Saunders C, Jensen R, Solomon GM, Vermeulen F, Kaiser A, Willmann S, Saleh S, Droebner K, Sandner P, Bear CE, Hoffmann A, Ratjen F, Rowe SM; Rio-CF Study Group. Riociguat for the treatment of Phe508del homozygous adults with cystic fibrosis. J Cyst Fibros 2021; 20:1018-25. doi: 10.1016/j.jcf.2021.07.015.

Di A, Brown ME, Deriy LV, Li C, Szeto FL, Chen Y, Huang P, Tong J, Naren AP, Bindokas V, Palfrey HC, Nelson DJ. CFTR regulates phagosome acidification in macrophages and alters bactericidal activity. Nat Cell Biol 2006;8:933-44. doi: 10.1038/ncb1456.

Donaldson SH, Solomon GM, Zeitlin PL, Flume PA, Casey A, McCoy K, Zemanick ET, Mandagere A, Troha JM, Shoemaker SA, Chmiel JF, Taylor-Cousar JL. Pharmacokinetics and safety of cavosonstat (N91115) in healthy and cystic fibrosis adults homozygous for F508DEL-CFTR. J Cyst Fibros 2017;16:371-9. doi: 10.1016/j.jcf.2017.01.009.

Donaldson SH, Laube BL, Corcoran TE, Bhambhvani P, Zeman K, Ceppe A, Zeitlin PL, Mogayzel PJ Jr, Boyle M, Locke LW, Myerburg MM, Pilewski JM, Flanagan B, Rowe SM, Bennett WD. Effect of ivacaftor on mucociliary clearance and clinical outcomes in cystic fibrosis patients with G551D-CFTR. JCI Insight 2018;3:e122695. doi: 10.1172/jci.insight.122695.

Donaldson SH, Laube BL, Mogayzel P, Corcoran TE, Pilewski JM, Ceppe A, Wu J, Bhambhvani PG, Ratjen F, Sagel SD, Clancy JP, Rowe SM, Bennett WD. Effect of lumacaftor-ivacaftor on mucociliary clearance and clinical outcomes in cystic fibrosis: Results from the PROSPECT MCC sub-study. J Cyst Fibros 2021:S1569-1993(21)00131-4. doi: 10.1016/j.jcf.2021.05.004.

Donaldson SH, Pilewski JM, Griese M, Cooke J, Viswanathan L, Tullis E, Davies JC, Lekstrom-Himes JA, Wang LT; VX11-661-101 Study Group. Tezacaftor/Ivacaftor in subjects with cystic fibrosis and F508del/F508del-CFTR or F508del/G551D-CFTR. Am J Respir Crit Care Med 2018;197:214-224. doi: 10.1164/rccm.201704-0717OC.

Drevinek P, Pressler T, Cipolli M, De Boeck K, Schwarz C, Bouisset F, Boff M, Henig N, Paquette-Lamontagne N, Montgomery S, Perquin J, Tomkinson N, den Hollander W, Elborn JS. Antisense oligonucleotide eluforsen is safe and improves respiratory symptoms in F508DEL cystic fibrosis. J Cyst Fibros 2020;19:99-107. doi: 10.1016/j.jcf.2019.05.014.

Duckers J, Lesher B, Thorat T, Lucas E, McGarry LJ, Chandarana K, De Iorio F. Real-world outcomes of ivacaftor treatment in people with cystic fibrosis: A systematic review. J Clin Med 2021;10:1527. doi: 10.3390/jcm10071527.

Eckford PD, Li C, Ramjeesingh M, Bear CE. Cystic fibrosis transmembrane conductance regulator (CFTR) potentiator VX-770 (ivacaftor) opens the defective channel gate of mutant CFTR in a phosphorylation-dependent but ATP-independent manner. J Biol Chem 2012; 287:36639-49. doi: 10.1074/jbc.M112.393637.

Edgeworth D, Keating D, Ellis M, Button B, Williams E, Clark D, Tierney A, Heritier S, Kotsimbos T, Wilson J. Improvement in exercise duration, lung function and well-being in G551D-cystic fibrosis patients: a double-blind, placebo-controlled, randomized, cross-over study with ivacaftor treatment. Clin Sci (Lond) 2017;131:2037-2045. doi: 10.1042/CS20170995

Einarsson GG, Ronan NJ, Mooney D, McGettigan C, Mullane D, NiChroinin M, Shanahan F, Murphy DM, McCarthy M, McCarthy Y, Eustace JA, Gilpin DF, Elborn JS, Plant BJ, Tunney MM. Extended-culture and culture-independent molecular analysis of the airway microbiota in cystic fibrosis following CFTR modulation with ivacaftor. J Cyst Fibros 2021;20:747-753. doi: 10.1016/j.jcf.2020.12.023.

Ejiofor LCK, Mathiesen IHM, Jensen-Fangel S, Olesen HV, Skov M, Philipsen LKD, Pedersen CL, Pressler T. Patients with cystic fibrosis and advanced lung disease benefit from lumacaftor/ivacaftor treatment. Pediatr Pulmonol 2020;55:3364-3370. doi: 10.1002/ppul.25059.

Estimation of the variation of exposure due to a drug-drug interaction—DDI-Predictor Academic version. (o. J.). Accessed on August 29th 2021, at https://www.ddi-predictor.org/predictor/ddi

Farinha CM, King-Underwood J, Sousa M, Correia AR, Henriques BJ, Roxo-Rosa M, Da Paula AC, Williams J, Hirst S, Gomes CM, Amaral MD. Revertants, low temperature, and correctors reveal the mechanism of F508del-CFTR rescue by VX-809 and suggest multiple agents for full correction. Chem Biol 2013;20:943-55. doi: 10.1016/j.chembiol.2013.06.004.

Flume PA, Biner RF, Downey DG, Brown C, Jain M, Fischer R, De Boeck K, Sawicki GS, Chang P, Paz-Diaz H, Rubin JL, Yang Y, Hu X, Pasta DJ, Millar SJ, Campbell D, Wang X, Ahluwalia N, Owen CA, Wainwright CE; VX14-661-110 study group. Long-term safety and efficacy of tezacaftor-ivacaftor in individuals with cystic fibrosis aged 12 years or older who are homozygous or heterozygous for Phe508del CFTR (EXTEND): an open-label extension study. Lancet Respir Med 2021;9:733-46. doi: 10.1016/S2213-2600(20)30510-5.

Flume PA, Liou TG, Borowitz DS, Li H, Yen K, Ordoñez CL, Geller DE; VX 08-770-104 Study Group. Ivacaftor in subjects with cystic fibrosis who are homozygous for the F508del-CFTR mutation. Chest 2012;142:718-724. doi: 10.1378/chest.11-2672.

Flume PA, Wainwright CE, Elizabeth Tullis D, Rodriguez S, Niknian M, Higgins M, Davies JC, Wagener JS. Recovery of lung function following a pulmonary exacerbation in patients with cystic fibrosis and the G551D-CFTR mutation treated with ivacaftor. J Cyst Fibros 2018;17:83-88. doi: 10.1016/j.jcf.2017.06.002.

Fortner CN, Seguin JM, Kay DM. Normal pancreatic function and false-negative CF newborn screen in a child born to a mother taking *CFTR* modulator therapy during pregnancy. J Cyst Fibros 2021;20:835–836.

Frost FJ, Nazareth DS, Charman SC, Winstanley C, Walshaw MJ. Ivacaftor is associated with reduced lung infection by key cystic fibrosis pathogens. A cohort study using national registry data. Ann Am Thorac Soc 2019; 16:1375-1382. doi: 10.1513/AnnalsATS.201902-122OC

Gardner AI, Haq IJ, Simpson AJ, Becker KA, Gallagher J, Saint-Criq V, Verdon B, Mavin E, Trigg A, Gray MA, Koulman A, McDonnell MJ, Fisher AJ, Kramer EL, Clancy JP, Ward C, Schuchman EH, Gulbins E, Brodlie M. Recombinant acid ceramidase reduces inflammation and infection in cystic fibrosis. Am J Respir Crit Care Med. 2020;202:1133-1145. doi: 10.1164/rccm.202001-0180OC.

Garg V, Shen J, Li C, Agarwal S, Gebre A, Robertson S, Huang J, Han L, Jiang L, Stephan K, Wang LT, Lekstrom-Himes J. Pharmacokinetic and drug-drug interaction profiles of the combination of Tezacaftor/Ivacaftor. Clin Transl Sci. 2019;12:267-275. doi: 10.1111/cts.12610.

Gavioli EM, Guardado N, Haniff F, Deiab N, Vider E. A current review of the safety of cystic fibrosis transmembrane conductance regulator modulators. J Clin Pharm Ther. 2021;46:286-294. doi: 10.1111/jcpt.13329.

Gelfond D, Heltshe S, Ma C, Rowe SM, Frederick C, Uluer A, Sicilian L, Konstan M, Tullis E, Roach RN, Griffin K, Joseloff E, Borowitz D. Impact of CFTR modulation on intestinal pH, motility, and clinical outcomes in patients with cystic fibrosis and the G551D mutation. Clin Transl Gastroenterol 2017; 8:e81. doi: 10.1038/ctg.2017.10.

Graeber SY, Boutin S, Wielpütz MO, Joachim C, Frey DL, Wege S, Sommerburg O, Kauczor HU, Stahl M, Dalpke AH, Mall MA. Effects of Lumacaftor-Ivacaftor on lung clearance index, magnetic resonance imaging, and airway microbiome in Phe508del homozygous patients with cystic fibrosis. Ann Am Thorac Soc. 2021;18: 971-980. doi: 10.1513/AnnalsATS

Graeber SY, Dopfer C, Naehrlich L, Gyulumyan L, Scheuermann H, Hirtz S, Wege S, Mairbäurl H, Dorda M, Hyde R, Bagheri-Hanson A, Rueckes-Nilges C, Fischer S, Mall MA, Tümmler B. Effects of Lumacaftor-Ivacaftor therapy on Cystic Fibrosis Transmembrane Conductance Regulator function in Phe508del homozygous patients with cystic fibrosis. Am J Respir Crit Care Med 2018;197:1433-42. doi: 10.1164/rccm.201710-1983 OC

Graeber SY, Hug MJ, Sommerburg O, Hirtz S, Hentschel J, Heinzmann A, Dopfer C, Schulz A, Mainz JG, Tümmler B, Mall MA. Intestinal current measurements detect activation of mutant CFTR in patients with cystic fibrosis with the G551D mutation treated with Ivacaftor. Am J Respir Crit Care Med 2015; 192:1252-5. doi: 10. 1164/rccm.201507-1271LE.

Graeber SY, Vitzthum C, Pallenberg ST, Naehrlich L, Stahl M, Rohrbach A, Drescher M, Minso R, Ringshausen FC, Rueckes-Nilges C, Klajda J, Berges J, Yu Y, Scheuermann H, Hirtz S, Sommerburg O, Dittrich AM, Tümmler B, Mall MA. Effects of Elexacaftor/Tezacaftor/Ivacaftor therapy on CFTR function in patients with cystic fibrosis and one or two *F508del* alleles. Am J Respir Crit Care Med. 2022;204:in press. doi: 10.1164/ rccm.202110-2249OC.

Gramegna A, Contarini M, Aliberti S, Casciaro R, Blasi F, Castellani C. From ivacaftor to triple combination: A systematic review of efficacy and safety of CFTR modulators in people with cystic fibrosis. Int J Mol Sci. 2020; 21:5882. doi: 10.3390/ijms21165882.

Granger E, Davies G, Keogh RH. Treatment patterns in people with cystic fibrosis: have they changed since the introduction of ivacaftor? J Cyst Fibros 2021:S1569-1993 (21)01355-2. doi: 10.1016/j.jcf.2021.08.014.

Green M, Lindgren N, Henderson A, Keith JD, Oden AM, Birket SE. Ivacaftor partially corrects airway inflammation in a humanized G551D rat. Am J Physiol Lung Cell Mol Physiol. 2021;320:L1093-L1100. doi: 10.1152/ ajplung.00082.2021.

Griese M, Costa S, Linnemann RW, Mall MA, McKone EF, Polineni D, Quon BS, Ringshausen FC, Taylor-Cousar JL, Withers NJ, Moskowitz SM, Daines CL. Safety and efficacy of Elexacaftor/Tezacaftor/Ivacaftor for 24 weeks or longer in people with cystic fibrosis and one or more F508del alleles: Interim results of an open-label phase 3 clinical trial. Am J Respir Crit Care Med 2021;203:381-5. doi: 10.1164/rccm.202008-3176LE.

Guerra L, D'Oria S, Favia M, Castellani S, Santostasi T, Polizzi AM, Mariggiò MA, Gallo C, Casavola V, Montemurro P, Leonetti G, Manca A, Conese M. CFTR-dependent chloride efflux in cystic fibrosis mononuclear cells is increased by ivacaftor therapy. Pediatr Pulmonol 2017;52:900-8. doi: 10.1002/ppul.23712.

Guhr Lee TN, Cholon DM, Quinney NL, Gentzsch M, Esther CR Jr. Accumulation and persistence of ivacaftor in airway epithelia with prolonged treatment. J Cyst Fibros 2020;19:746-751. doi: 10.1016/j.jcf.2020.04.010.

Guimbellot J, Solomon GM, Baines A, Heltshe SL, Van Dalfsen J, Joseloff E, Sagel SD, Rowe SM; GOALe(2) Investigators. Effectiveness of ivacaftor in cystic fibrosis patients with non-G551D gating mutations. J Cyst Fibros 2019;18:102-109. doi: 10.1016/j.jcf.2018.04.004.

Guimbellot JS, Baines A, Paynter A, Heltshe SL, Van Dalfsen J, Jain M, Rowe SM, Sagel SD; GOAL-e2 Investigators. Long term clinical effectiveness of ivacaftor in people with the G551D CFTR mutation. J Cyst Fibros 2021;20:213-219. doi: 10.1016/j.jcf.2020.11.008.

Haggie PM, Verkman AS. Cystic fibrosis transmembrane conductance regulator-independent phagosomal acidification in macrophages. J Biol Chem. 2007;282: 31422-8. doi: 10.1074/jbc.M705296200.

Han ST, Rab A, Pellicore MJ, Davis EF, McCague AF, Evans TA, Joynt AT, Lu Z, Cai Z, Raraigh KS, Hong JS, Sheppard DN, Sorscher EJ, Cutting GR. Residual function of cystic fibrosis mutants predicts response to small molecule CFTR modulators. JCI Insight 2018;3:e121159. doi: 10.1172/jci.insight.121159.

Hardisty GR, Law SM, Carter S, Grogan B, Singh PK, McKone EF, Gray RD. Ivacaftor modifies cystic fibrosis neutrophil phenotype in subjects with R117H residual function CFTR mutations. Eur Respir J. 2021;57: 2002161. doi: 10.1183/13993003.02161-2020.

Harris JK, Wagner BD, Zemanick ET, Robertson CE, Stevens MJ, Heltshe SL, Rowe SM, Sagel SD. Changes in airway microbiome and inflammation with ivacaftor treatment in patients with cystic fibrosis and the G551D mutation. Ann Am Thorac Soc 2020;17:212-220. doi: 10.1513/ AnnalsATS.201907-493OC.

He L, Kota P, Aleksandrov AA, Cui L, Jensen T, Dokholyan NV, Riordan JR. Correctors of ΔF508 CFTR restore global conformational maturation without thermally stabilizing the mutant protein. FASEB J. 2013; 27:536-45. doi: 10.1096/fj.12-216119.

Hebestreit H, Sauer-Heilborn A, Fischer R, Käding M, Mainz JG. Effects of ivacaftor on severely ill patients with cystic fibrosis carrying a G551D mutation. J Cyst Fibros 2013;12:599-603. doi: 10.1016/j.jcf.2013.05.006.

Heijerman HGM, McKone EF, Downey DG, Van Braeckel E, Rowe SM, Tullis E, Mall MA, Welter JJ, Ramsey BW, McKee CM, Marigowda G, Moskowitz SM, Waltz D, Sosnay PR, Simard C, Ahluwalia N, Xuan F, Zhang Y, Taylor-Cousar JL, McCoy KS; VX17-445-103 Trial Group. Efficacy and safety of the elexacaftor plus tezacaftor plus ivacaftor combination regimen in people with cystic fibrosis homozygous for the F508del mutation: a double-blind, randomised, phase 3 trial. Lancet 2019;394:1940-8. doi: 10.1016/S0140-6736(19)32597-8.

Heltshe SL, Mayer-Hamblett N, Burns JL, Khan U, Baines A, Ramsey BW, Rowe SM; GOAL (the G551D Observation-AL) Investigators of the Cystic Fibrosis Foundation Therapeutics Development Network. *Pseudomonas aeruginosa* in cystic fibrosis patients with G551D-CFTR treated with ivacaftor. Clin Infect Dis 2015;60:703-12. doi: 10.1093/cid/ciu944.

Heltshe SL, Rowe SM, Skalland M, Baines A, Jain M; GOAL Investigators of the Cystic Fibrosis Foundation Therapeutics Development Network. Ivacaftor-treated patients with cystic fibrosis derive long-term benefit despite no short-term clinical improvement. Am J Respir Crit Care Med 2018;197:1483-1486. doi: 10.1164/rccm.201710-2046LE.

Heo S, Young DC, Safirstein J, Antell MH, Diloreto S, Rotolo SM. Mental status changes during elexacaftor/tezacaftor / ivacaftor therapy. J Cyst Fibros 2021; https://doi.org/10.1016/ j.jcf.2021.10.002.

Higgins M, Volkova N, Moy K, Marshall BC, Bilton D. Real-world outcomes among patients with cystic fibrosis treated with Ivacaftor: 2012-2016 experience. Pulm Ther 2020;6:141-149. doi: 10.1007/s41030-020-00115-8.

Hisert KB, Heltshe SL, Pope C, Jorth P, Wu X, Edwards RM, Radey M, Accurso FJ, Wolter DJ, Cooke G, Adam RJ, Carter S, Grogan B, Launspach JL, Donnelly SC, Gallagher CG, Bruce JE, Stoltz DA, Welsh MJ, Hoffman LR, McKone EF, Singh PK. Restoring Cystic Fibrosis Transmembrane Conductance Regulator function reduces airway bacteria and inflammation in people with cystic fibrosis and chronic lung infections. Am J Respir Crit Care Med 2017;195:1617-1628. doi: 10.1164/rccm.201609-1954OC.

Hisert KB, Birkland TP, Schoenfelt KQ, Long ME, Grogan B, Carter S, Liles WC, McKone EF, Becker L, Manicone AM. Ivacaftor decreases monocyte sensitivity to interferon-γ in people with cystic fibrosis. ERJ Open Res 2020;6:00318-2019. doi: 10.1183/23120541.00318-2019.

Hoppe JE, Chilvers M, Ratjen F, McNamara JJ, Owen CA, Tian S, Zahigian R, Cornell AG, McColley SA. Long-term safety of lumacaftor-ivacaftor in children aged 2-5 years with cystic fibrosis homozygous for the F508del-CFTR mutation: a multicentre, phase 3, open-label, extension study. Lancet Respir Med 2021;9:977-988. doi: 10.1016/S2213-2600(21)00069-2.

Hubert D, Dehillotte C, Munck A, David V, Baek J, Mely L, Dominique S, Ramel S, Danner Boucher I, Lefeuvre S, Reynaud Q, Colomb-Jung V, Bakouboula P, Lemonnier L. Retrospective observational study of French patients with cystic fibrosis and a Gly551Asp-CFTR mutation after 1 and 2 years of treatment with ivacaftor in a real-world setting. J Cyst Fibros 2018;17:89-95. doi: 10.1016/j.jcf.2017.07.001.

Hubert D, Marguet C, Benichou J, DeSouza C, Payen-Champenois C, Kinnman N, Chandarana K, Munck A, Fajac I; BRIO Study Group. Real-world long-term Ivacaftor for cystic fibrosis in France: Clinical effectiveness and healthcare resource utilization. Pulm Ther 2021; 7:455-468. doi: 10.1007/s41030-021-00158-5

Hudson RP, Dawson JE, Chong PA, Yang Z, Millen L, Thomas PJ, Brouillette CG, Forman-Kay JD. Direct binding of the corrector VX-809 to human CFTR NBD1: Evidence of an allosteric coupling between the binding site and the NBD1:CL4 interface. Mol Pharmacol 2017; 92:124-135. doi: 10.1124/ mol.117.108373.

Indiana University School of Medicine & Division of Clinical Pharmacology. (o. J.). CYTOCHROME P450 DRUG INTERACTION TABLE - Drug Interactions. Drug Interactions Flockhart Table™. Accessed on October 10th 2021, at https://drug-interactions.medicine.iu.edu/MainTable.aspx

Jani M, Ambrus C, Magnan R, Jakab KT, Beéry E, Zolnerciks JK, Krajcsi P. Structure and function of BCRP, a broad specificity transporter of xenobiotics and endobiotics. Arch Toxicol. 2014;88:1205-48. doi: 10.1007/s00204-014-1224-8.

Jarosz-Griffiths HH, Scambler T, Wong CH, Lara-Reyna S, Holbrook J, Martinon F, Savic S, Whitaker P, Etherington C, Spoletini G, Clifton I, Mehta A, McDermott MF, Peckham D. Different CFTR modulator combinations downregulate inflammation differently in cystic fibrosis. Elife 2020;9:e54556. doi: 10.7554/eLife.54556.

Jih KY, Hwang TC. Vx-770 potentiates CFTR function by promoting decoupling between the gating cycle and ATP hydrolysis cycle. Proc Natl Acad Sci U S A 2013;110:4404-9. doi: 10.1073/ pnas.1215982110.

Kawala CR, Ma X, Sykes J, Stanojevic S, Coriati A, Stephenson AL. Real-world use of ivacaftor in Canada: A retrospective analysis using the Canadian Cystic Fibrosis Registry. J Cyst Fibros 2021;20:1040-1045. doi: 10.1016/j.jcf.2021.03.008.

Keating D, Marigowda G, Burr L, Daines C, Mall MA, McKone EF, Ramsey BW, Rowe SM, Sass LA, Tullis E, McKee CM, Moskowitz SM, Robertson S, Savage J, Simard C, Van Goor F, Waltz D, Xuan F, Young T, Taylor-Cousar JL; VX16-445-001 Study Group. VX-445-Tezacaftor-Ivacaftor in patients with cystic fibrosis and one or two Phe508del alleles. N Engl J Med 2018;379:1612-1620. doi: 10.1056/NEJMoa1807120.

Kerem B, Rommens JM, Buchanan JA, Markiewicz D, Cox TK, Chakravarti A, Buchwald M, Tsui LC. Identification of the cystic fibrosis gene: genetic analysis. Science 1989;245:1073-80. doi: 10.1126/science.2570460.

Kim J, Farahmand M, Dunn C, Milla CE, Horii RI, Thomas EAC, Moss RB, Wine JJ. Sweat rate analysis of ivacaftor potentiation of CFTR in non-CF adults. Sci Rep 2018;8:16233. doi: 10.1038/s41598-018-34308-8.

Kim SO, Corey M, Stephenson AL, Strug LJ. Reference percentiles of FEV1 for the Canadian cystic fibrosis population: comparisons across time and countries. Thorax. 2018;73:446-450. doi: 10.1136/thoraxjnl-2017-210899.

King SJ, Tierney AC, Edgeworth D, Keating D, Williams E, Kotsimbos T, Button BM, Wilson JW. Body composition and weight changes after ivacaftor treatment in adults with cystic fibrosis carrying the G551 D cystic fibrosis transmembrane conductance regulator mutation: A double-blind, placebo-controlled, randomized, crossover study with open-label extension. Nutrition 2021;85: 111124. doi: 10.1016/j.nut.2020.111124.

Kleizen B, van Willigen M, Mijnders M, Peters F, Grudniewska M, Hillenaar T, Thomas A, Kooijman L, Peters KW, Frizzell R, van der Sluijs P, Braakman I. Co-translational folding of the first transmembrane domain of ABC-transporter CFTR is supported by assembly with the first cytosolic domain. J Mol Biol 2021;433:166955. doi: 10.1016/j.jmb.2021.166955.

Konstan MW, McKone EF, Moss RB, Marigowda G, Tian S, Waltz D, Huang X, Lubarsky B, Rubin J, Millar SJ, Pasta DJ, Mayer-Hamblett N, Goss CH, Morgan W, Sawicki GS. Assessment of safety and efficacy of long-term treatment with combination lumacaftor and ivacaftor therapy in patients with cystic fibrosis homozygous for the F508del-CFTR mutation (PROGRESS): a phase 3, extension study. Lancet Respir Med 2017;5:107-118. doi: 10.1016/S2213-2600(16)30427-1.

Kopeikin Z, Yuksek Z, Yang HY, Bompadre SG. Combined effects of VX-770 and VX-809 on several functional abnormalities of F508del-CFTR channels. J Cyst Fibros 2014;13:508-14. doi: 10.1016/j.jcf.2014.04.003.

Krainer G, Schenkel M, Hartmann A, Ravamehr-Lake D, Deber CM, Schlierf M. CFTR transmembrane segments are impaired in their conformational adaptability by a pathogenic loop mutation and dynamically stabilized by Lumacaftor. J Biol Chem 2020;295:1985-91. doi: 0.1074/jbc.AC119.011360.

Kristensen MI, de Winter-de Groot KM, Berkers G, Chu MLJN, Arp K, Ghijsen S, Heijerman HGM, Arets HGM, Majoor CJ, Janssens HM, van der Meer R, Bogaert D, van der Ent CK. Individual and group response of treatment with Ivacaftor on airway and gut microbiota in people with CF and a S1251N mutation. J Pers Med 2021;11: 350. doi: 10.3390/jpm11050350.

Langron E, Prins S, Vergani P. Potentiation of the cystic fibrosis transmembrane conductance regulator by VX-770 involves stabilization of the pre-hydrolytic, O_1 state. Br J Pharmacol 2018; 175:3990-4002. doi: 10.1111/bph.14475.

Laselva O, Bartlett C, Gunawardena TNA, Ouyang H, Eckford PDW, Moraes TJ, Bear CE, Gonska T. Rescue of multiple class II CFTR mutations by elexacaftor+tezacaftor+ivacaftor mediated in part by the dual activities of elexacaftor as both corrector and potentiator. Eur Respir J 2021;57:2002774. doi: 10.1183/13993003.02774-2020

Laselva O, Molinski S, Casavola V, Bear CE. Correctors of the major cystic fibrosis mutant interact through membrane-spanning domains. Mol Pharmacol 2018;93: 612-618. doi: 10.1124/ mol.118.111799.

Laselva O, Qureshi Z, Zeng ZW, Petrotchenko EV, Ramjeesingh M, Hamilton CM, Huan LJ, Borchers CH, Pomès R, Young R, Bear CE. Identification of binding sites for ivacaftor on the cystic fibrosis transmembrane conductance regulator. iScience 2021;24:102542. doi: 10.1016/j.isci.2021.102542

Liessi N, Pesce E, Braccia C, Bertozzi SM, Giraudo A, Bandiera T, Pedemonte N, Armirotti A. Distinctive lipid signatures of bronchial epithelial cells associated with cystic fibrosis drugs, including Trikafta. JCI Insight 2020; 5:e138722. doi: 10.1172/jci.insight.138722.

Liu F, Zhang Z, Levit A, Levring J, Touhara KK, Shoichet BK, Chen J. Structural identification of a hotspot on CFTR for potentiation. Science 2019;364:1184-1188. doi: 10.1126/science.aaw7611

Loo TW, Clarke DM. Corrector VX-809 promotes interactions between cytoplasmic loop one and the first nucleotide-binding domain of CFTR. Biochem Pharmacol 2017;136:24-31. doi: 10.1016/j.bcp.2017.03.020.

Loukou I, Moustaki M, Plyta M, Douros K. Longitudinal changes in lung function following initiation of lumacaftor/ivacaftor combination. J Cyst Fibros 2020;19:534-539. doi: 10.1016/j.jcf.2019.09.009.

Lowry S, Mogayzel PJ, Oshima K, Karnsakul W. Drug-induced liver injury from elexacaftor/ivacaftor/ tezacaftor. J Cyst Fibros 2021:S1569-1993(21)01297-2. doi: 10.1016/j.jcf.2021.07.001.

Mainz JG, Arnold C, Wittstock K, Hipler UC, Lehmann T, Zagoya C, Duckstein F, Ellemunter H, Hentschel J. Ivacaftor reduces inflammatory mediators in upper airway lining fluid from cystic fibrosis patients with a G551D mutation: Serial non-invasive home-based collection of upper airway lining fluid. Front Immunol 2021;12:642180. doi: 10.3389/fimmu.2021.642180.

Masson A, Schneider-Futschik EK, Baatallah N, Nguyen-Khoa T, Girodon E, Hatton A, Flament T, Le Bourgeois M, Chedevergne F, Bailly C, Kyrilli S, Achimastos D, Hinzpeter A, Edelman A, Sermet-Gaudelus I. Predictive factors for lumacaftor/ivacaftor clinical response. J Cyst Fibros. 2019;18:368-374. doi: 10.1016/j.jcf.2018.12.011.

Mayer-Hamblett N, Nichols DP, Odem-Davis K, Riekert KA, Sawicki GS, Donaldson SH, Ratjen F, Konstan MW, Simon N, Rosenbluth DB, Retsch-Bogart G, Clancy JP, VanDalfsen JM, Buckingham R, Gifford AH. Evaluating the impact of stopping chronic therapies after modulator drug therapy in cystic fibrosis: The SIMPLIFY clinical trial study design. Ann Am Thorac Soc 2021;18:1397-1405. doi: 10.1513/AnnalsATS.202010-1336SD.

McColley SA, Konstan MW, Ramsey BW, Stuart Elborn J, Boyle MP, Wainwright CE, Waltz D, Vera-Llonch M, Marigowda G, Jiang JG, Rubin JL. Lumacaftor/Ivacaftor reduces pulmonary exacerbations in patients irrespective of initial changes in FEV1. J Cyst Fibros 2019;18:94-101. doi: 10.1016/ j.jcf.2018.07.011.

McGarry ME, Illek B, Ly NP, Zlock L, Olshansky S, Moreno C, Finkbeiner WE, Nielson DW. In vivo and in vitro ivacaftor response in cystic fibrosis patients with residual CFTR function: N-of-1 studies. Pediatr Pulmonol 2017;52:472-479. doi: 10.1002/ppul.23659.

McKone EF, Borowitz D, Drevinek P, Griese M, Konstan MW, Wainwright C, Ratjen F, Sermet-Gaudelus I, Plant B, Munck A, Jiang Y, Gilmartin G, Davies JC; VX08-770-105 (PERSIST) Study Group. Long-term safety and efficacy of ivacaftor in patients with cystic fibrosis who have the Gly551Asp-CFTR mutation: a phase 3, open-label extension study (PERSIST). Lancet Respir Med. 2014; 2:902-910. doi: 10.1016/S2213-2600(14)70218-8.

McKone EF, DiMango EA, Sutharsan S, Barto TL, Campbell D, Ahluwalia N, Higgins M, Owen CA, Tullis E. A phase 3, randomized, double-blind, parallel-group study to evaluate tezacaftor/ivacaftor in people with cystic fibrosis heterozygous for F508del-CFTR and a gating mutation. J Cyst Fibros 2021; 20:234-42. doi: 10.1016/ j.jcf.2020.11.003.

McLean KJ, Munro AW. (2018). Cytochrome P450 (cyp). In S. Choi (Eds.): Encyclopedia of signaling molecules 2018, pp. 1288–1305. Springer International Publishing, New York.

McNamara JJ, McColley SA, Marigowda G, Liu F, Tian S, Owen CA, Stiles D, Li C, Waltz D, Wang LT, Sawicki GS. Safety, pharmacokinetics, and pharmacodynamics of lumacaftor and ivacaftor combination therapy in children aged 2-5 years with cystic fibrosis homozygous for F508del-CFTR: an open-label phase 3 study. Lancet Respir Med 2019;7:325-335. doi: 10.1016/S2213-2600 (18)30460-0.

Merkert S, Schubert M, Olmer R, Engels L, Radetzki S, Veltman M, Scholte BJ, Zöllner J, Pedemonte N, Galietta LJV, von Kries JP, Martin U. High-throughput screening for modulators of CFTR activity based on genetically engineered cystic fibrosis disease-specific iPSCs. Stem Cell Reports 2019;12:1389-1403. doi: 10.1016/j.stemcr.2019. 04.014.

Mehta Z, Kamal KM, Miller R, Covvey JR, Giannetti V. Adherence to cystic fibrosis transmembrane conductance regulator (CFTR) modulators: analysis of a national specialty pharmacy database. J Drug Assess 2021; 10:62-67. doi: 10.1080/21556660.2021.1912352.

Middleton PG, Mall MA, Døevínek P, Lands LC, Mc Kone EF, Polineni D, Ramsey BW, Taylor-Cousar JL, Tullis E, Vermeulen F, Marigowda G, McKee CM, Moskowitz SM, Nair N, Savage J, Simard C, Tian S, Waltz D, Xuan F, Rowe SM, Jain R; VX17-445-102 Study Group. Elexacaftor-Tezacaftor-Ivacaftor for cystic fibrosis with a single Phe508del allele. N Engl J Med 2019;381:1809-19. doi: 10.1056/NEJMoa1908639.

Milla CE, Ratjen F, Marigowda G, Liu F, Waltz D, Rosenfeld M; VX13-809-011 Part B Investigator Group. Lumacaftor/Ivacaftor in patients aged 6-11 years with cystic fibrosis and homozygous for F508del-CFTR. Am J Respir Crit Care Med 2017;195:912-920. doi: 10.1164/ rccm.201608-1754OC

Moheet A, Beisang D, Zhang L, Sagel SD, VanDalfsen JM, Heltshe SL, Frederick C, Mann M, Antos N, Billings J, Rowe SM, Moran A; PROSPECT Investigators of the Cystic Fibrosis Foundation Therapeutics Development Network. Lumacaftor/ivacaftor therapy fails to increase insulin secretion in F508del/F508del CF patients. J Cyst Fibros 2021;20:333-38. doi: 10.1016/j.jcf.2020.09.001.

Molinski SV, Shahani VM, Subramanian AS, Mac Kinnon SS, Woollard G, Laforet M, Laselva O, Morayniss LD, Bear CE, Windemuth A. Comprehensive mapping of cystic fibrosis mutations to CFTR protein identifies mutation clusters and molecular docking predicts corrector binding site. Proteins 2018;86:833-843. doi: 10.1002/prot.25496.

Morrison CB, Shaffer KM, Araba KC, Markovetz MR, Wykoff JA, Quinney NL, Hao S, Delion MF, Flen AL, Morton LC, Liao J, Hill DB, Drumm ML, O'Neal WK, Kesimer M, Gentzsch M, Ehre C. Treatment of cystic fibrosis airway cells with CFTR modulators reverses aberrant mucus properties via hydration. Eur Respir J 2021: 2100185. doi: 10.1183/13993003.00185-2021.

Moss RB, Flume PA, Elborn JS, Cooke J, Rowe SM, McColley SA, Rubenstein RC, Higgins M; VX11-770-110 (KONDUCT) Study Group. Efficacy and safety of ivacaftor in patients with cystic fibrosis who have an Arg117His-CFTR mutation: a double-blind, randomised controlled trial. Lancet Respir Med 2015;3: 524-33. doi: 10.1016/S2213-2600(15)00201-5.

Munck A, Kerem E, Ellemunter H, Campbell D, Wang LT, Ahluwalia N, Owen CA, Wainwright C. Tezacaftor/ ivacaftor in people with cystic fibrosis heterozygous for minimal function CFTR mutations. J Cyst Fibros 2020; 19:962-68. doi: 10.1016/j.jcf.2020.04.015.

Neerincx AH, Whiteson K, Phan JL, Brinkman P, Abdel-Aziz MI, Weersink EJM, Altenburg J, Majoor CJ, Maitland-van der Zee AH, Bos LDJ. Lumacaftor/ivacaftor changes the lung microbiome and metabolome in cystic fibrosis patients. ERJ Open Res 2021;7:00731-2020. doi: 10.1183/23120541.00731-2020.

Nichols AL, Davies JC, Jones D, Carr SB. Restoration of exocrine pancreatic function in older children with cystic fibrosis on ivacaftor. Paediatr Respir Rev 2020;35:99-102. doi: 10.1016/j.prrv.2020.04.003.

Nichols DP, Donaldson SH, Frederick CA, Freedman SD, Gelfond D, Hoffman LR, Kelly A, Narkewicz MR, Pittman JE, Ratjen F, Sagel SD, Rosenfeld M, Schwarzenberg SJ, Singh PK, Solomon GM, Stalvey MS, Kirby S, VanDalfsen JM, Clancy JP, Rowe SM. PROMISE: Working with the CF community to understand emerging clinical and research needs for those treated with highly effective CFTR modulator therapy. J Cyst Fibros 2021a;20:205-212. doi: 10.1016/j.jcf.2021.02.003.

Nichols DP, Paynter AC, Heltshe SL, Donaldson SH, Frederick CA, Freedman SD, Gelfond D, Hoffman LR, Kelly A, Narkewicz MR, Pittman JE, Ratjen F, Rosenfeld M, Sagel SD, Schwarzenberg SJ, Singh PK, Solomon GM, Stalvey MS, Clancy JP, Kirby S, Van Dalfsen JM, Kloster MH, Rowe SM; PROMISE Study Group. Clinical effectiveness of Elexacaftor/Tezacaftor/Ivacaftor in people with cystic fibrosis. Am J Respir Crit Care Med. 2021b Nov 16. doi: 10.1164/rccm.202108-1986OC.

Nick JA, St Clair C, Jones MC, Lan L, Higgins M; VX12-770-113 Study Team. Ivacaftor in cystic fibrosis with residual function: Lung function results from an N-of-1 study. J Cyst Fibros 2020;19:91-8. doi: 10.1016/j.jcf.2019.09.013.

Nietert MM, Vinhoven L, Auer F, Hafkemeyer S, Stanke F. Comprehensive analysis of chemical structures that have been tested as CFTR activating substances in a publicly available database CandActCFTR. Front Pharmacol. 2021, 12:689205 doi: https://doi.org/10. 3389/fphar.2021.689205.

O'Connor KE, Goodwin DL, NeSmith A, Garcia B, Mingora C, Ladores SL, Rowe SM, Krick S, Solomon GM. Elexacaftor/tezacaftor/ivacaftor resolves subfertility in females with CF: A two center case series. J Cyst Fibros 2021;20:399-401. doi: 10.1016/j.jcf.2020.12.011.

Okiyoneda T, Veit G, Dekkers JF, Bagdany M, Soya N, Xu H, Roldan A, Verkman AS, Kurth M, Simon A, Hegedus T, Beekman JM, Lukacs GL. Mechanism-based corrector combination restores ΔF508-CFTR folding and function. Nat Chem Biol 2013;9:444-54. doi: 10.1038/nchembio.1253.

Oliver KE, Rauscher R, Mijnders M, Wang W, Wolpert MJ, Maya J, Sabusap CM, Kesterson RA, Kirk KL, Rab A, Braakman I, Hong JS, Hartman JL 4th, Ignatova Z, Sorscher EJ. Slowing ribosome velocity restores folding and function of mutant CFTR. J Clin Invest 2019;129: 5236-5253. doi: 10.1172/JCI124282.

Pallenberg ST, Junge S, Ringshausen FC, Sauer-Heilborn A, Hansen G, Dittrich AM, Tümmler B, Nietert M. CFTR modulation with elexacaftor-tezacaftor-ivacaftor in people with cystic fibrosis assessed by the β-adrenergic sweat rate assay. J Cyst Fibros 2021;21; doi.org/10.1016/j.cf.2021.10.005.

Pedemonte N, Bertozzi F, Caci E, Sorana F, Di Fruscia P, Tomati V, Ferrera L, Rodríguez-Gimeno A, Berti F, Pesce E, Sondo E, Gianotti A, Scudieri P, Bandiera T, Galietta LJV. Discovery of a picomolar potency pharmacological corrector of the mutant CFTR chloride channel. Sci Adv 2020;6:eaay9669. doi: 10.1126/sciadv.aay9669.

Pedemonte N, Lukacs GL, Du K, Caci E, Zegarra-Moran O, Galietta LJ, Verkman AS. Small-molecule correctors of defective DeltaF508-CFTR cellular processing identified by high-throughput screening. J Clin Invest 2005; 115:2564-71. doi: 10.1172/JCI24898.

Peleg AY, Choo JM, Langan KM, Edgeworth D, Keating D, Wilson J, Rogers GB, Kotsimbos T. Antibiotic exposure and interpersonal variance mask the effect of ivacaftor on respiratory microbiota composition. J Cyst Fibros.2018;17:50-6. doi: 10.1016/j.jcf.2017.08.002.

Pesci E, Bettinetti L, Fanti P, Galietta LJ, La Rosa S, Magnoni L, Pedemonte N, Sardone GL, Maccari L. Novel hits in the correction of ΔF508-Cystic Fibrosis Transmembrane Conductance Regulator (CFTR) protein: Synthesis, pharmacological, and ADME evaluation of Tetrahydropyrido[4,3-d]pyrimidines for the potential treatment of cystic fibrosis. J Med Chem 2015;58: 9697-711. doi: 10.1021/acs.jmedchem.5b00771.

Phuan PW, Veit G, Tan J, Roldan A, Finkbeiner WE, Lukacs GL, Verkman AS. Synergy-based small-molecule screen using a human lung epithelial cell line yields ΔF508-CFTR correctors that augment VX-809 maximal efficacy. Mol Pharmacol 2014;86:42-51. doi: 10.1124/mol.114.092478.

Phuan PW, Veit G, Tan JA, Finkbeiner WE, Lukacs GL, Verkman AS. Potentiators of defective ΔF508-CFTR gating that do not interfere with corrector action. Mol Pharmacol 2015;88:791-9. doi: 10.1124/mol.115.099689.

Pilewski JM, De Boeck K, Nick JA, Tian S, DeSouza C, Higgins M, Moss RB. Long-term Ivacaftor in people aged 6 years and older with cystic fibrosis with Ivacaftor-responsive mutations. Pulm Ther 2020;6:303-13. doi: 10.1007/s41030-020-00129-2

Popowicz N, Wood J, Tai A, Morey S, Mulrennan S. Immediate effects of lumacaftor/ivacaftor administration on lung function in patients with severe cystic fibrosis lung disease. J Cyst Fibros. 2017; 16:392-394. doi: 10.1016/j.jcf.2017.02.009.

Pranke IM, Hatton A, Simonin J, Jais JP, Le Pimpec-Barthes F, Carsin A, Bonnette P, Fayon M, Stremler-Le Bel N, Grenet D, Thumerel M, Mazenq J, Urbach V, Mesbahi M, Girodon-Boulandet E, Hinzpeter A, Edelman A, Sermet-Gaudelus I. Correction of CFTR function in nasal epithelial cells from cystic fibrosis patients predicts improvement of respiratory function by CFTR modulators. Sci Rep. 2017;7:7375. doi: 10.1038/s41598-017-07504-1.

Pranke I, Hatton A, Masson A, Flament T, Le Bourgeois M, Chedevergne F, Bailly C, Urbach V, Hinzpeter A, Edelman A, Sermet-Gaudelus I. Might brushed nasal cells be a surrogate for CFTR modulator clinical response? Am J Respir Crit Care Med 2019;199:123-126. doi: 10.1164/rccm.201808-1436LE.

Pugh RN, Murray-Lyon IM, Dawson JL, Pietroni MC, Williams R. Transection of the oesophagus for bleeding oesophageal varices. Br J Surg. 1973;60:646-9. doi: 10.1002/bjs.1800600817.

Putman MS, Greenblatt LB, Bruce M, Joseph T, Lee H, Sawicki G, Uluer A, Sicilian L, Neuringer I, Gordon CM, Bouxsein ML, Finkelstein JS. The effects of Ivacaftor on bone density and microarchitecture in children and adults with cystic fibrosis. J Clin Endocrinol Metab 2021; 106:e1248-e1261. doi: 10.1210/clinem/dgaa890.

Quittner AL, Buu A, Messer MA, Modi AC, Watrous M. Development and validation of The Cystic Fibrosis Questionnaire in the United States: a health-related quality-of-life measure for cystic fibrosis. Chest. 2005; 128:2347-54. doi: 10.1378/chest.128.4.2347.

Ramalho AS, Fürstová E, Vonk AM, Ferrante M, Verfaillie C, Dupont L, Boon M, Proesmans M, Beekman JM, Sarouk I, Vazquez Cordero C, Vermeulen F, De Boeck K; Belgian Organoid Project. Correction of CFTR function in intestinal organoids to guide treatment of cystic fibrosis. Eur Respir J. 2021;57:1902426. doi: 10.1183/13993003.02426-2019.

Ramsey BW, Davies J, McElvaney NG, Tullis E, Bell SC, Døevínek P, Griese M, McKone EF, Wainwright CE, Konstan MW, Moss R, Ratjen F, Sermet-Gaudelus I, Rowe SM, Dong Q, Rodriguez S, Yen K, Ordoñez C, Elborn JS; VX08-770-102 Study Group. A CFTR potentiator in patients with cystic fibrosis and the G551D mutation. N Engl J Med 2011;365:1663-72. doi: 10.1056/NEJMoa1105185.

Ratjen F, Hug C, Marigowda G, Tian S, Huang X, Stanojevic S, Milla CE, Robinson PD, Waltz D, Davies JC; VX14-809-109 investigator group. Efficacy and safety of lumacaftor and ivacaftor in patients aged 6-11 years with cystic fibrosis homozygous for F508del-CFTR: a randomised, placebo-controlled phase 3 trial. Lancet Respir Med 2017;5:557-567. doi: 10.1016/S2213-2600(17)30215-1.

Reix P, Tatopoulos A, Ioan I, Le Bourgeois M, Bui S, Choukroun ML, Bessaci-Kabouya K, Gerardin M, Bokov P, Da Silva J, Paillasseur JL, Burgel PR; French Cystic Fibrosis Reference Network study group. Real-world assessment of LCI following lumacaftor-ivacaftor initiation in adolescents and adults with cystic fibrosis. J Cyst Fibros 2021:S1569-1993(21)01286-8. doi: 10.1016/j.jcf.2021.06.002.

Ren HY, Grove DE, De La Rosa O, Houck SA, Sopha P, Van Goor F, Hoffman BJ, Cyr DM. VX-809 corrects folding defects in cystic fibrosis transmembrane conductance regulator protein through action on membrane-spanning domain 1. Mol Biol Cell 2013;24:3016-24. doi: 10.1091/mbc.E13-05-0240

Reznikov LR, Abou Alaiwa MH, Dohrn CL, Gansemer ND, Diekema DJ, Stoltz DA, Welsh MJ. Antibacterial properties of the CFTR potentiator ivacaftor. J Cyst Fibros 2014;13:515-9. doi: 10.1016/j.jcf.2014.02.004.

Rosenfeld M, Cunningham S, Harris WT, Lapey A, Regelmann WE, Sawicki GS, Southern KW, Chilvers M, Higgins M, Tian S, Cooke J, Davies JC; KLIMB study group. An open-label extension study of ivacaftor in children with CF and a CFTR gating mutation initiating treatment at age 2-5 years (KLIMB). J Cyst Fibros 2019; 18:838-43. doi: 10.1016/j.jcf.2019.03.009.

Rosenfeld M, Wainwright CE, Higgins M, Wang LT, McKee C, Campbell D, Tian S, Schneider J, Cunningham S, Davies JC; ARRIVAL study group. Ivacaftor treatment of cystic fibrosis in children aged 12 to <24 months and with a CFTR gating mutation (ARRIVAL): a phase 3 single-arm study. Lancet Respir Med 2018;6:545-553. doi: 10.1016/S2213-2600(18)30202-9.

Rowe SM, Heltshe SL, Gonska T, Donaldson SH, Borowitz D, Gelfond D, Sagel SD, Khan U, Mayer-Hamblett N, Van Dalfsen JM, Joseloff E, Ramsey BW; GOAL Investigators of the Cystic Fibrosis Foundation Therapeutics Development Network. Clinical mechanism of the cystic fibrosis transmembrane conductance regulator potentiator ivacaftor in G551D-mediated cystic fibrosis. Am J Respir Crit Care Med 2014;190:175-84. doi: 10.1164/rccm.201404-0703OC.

Rowe SM, Daines C, Ringshausen FC, Kerem E, Wilson J, Tullis E, Nair N, Simard C, Han L, Ingenito EP, McKee C, Lekstrom-Himes J, Davies JC. Tezacaftor-Ivacaftor in residual-function heterozygotes with cystic fibrosis. N Engl J Med 2017;377:2024-35. doi: 10.1056/NEJMoa1709847.

Rubin JL, O'Callaghan L, Pelligra C, Konstan MW, Ward A, Ishak JK, Chandler C, Liou TG. Modeling long-term health outcomes of patients with cystic fibrosis homozygous for F508del-CFTR treated with lumacaftor/ivacaftor. Ther Adv Respir Dis 2019;13:1753466618820186. doi: 10.1177/ 1753466618820186.

Safirstein J, Grant JJ, Clausen E, Savant D, Dezube R, Hong G. Biliary disease and cholecystectomy after initiation of elexacaftor/ivacaftor/tezacaftor in adults with cystic fibrosis. J Cyst Fibros 2021; 20:506-510. doi: 10.1016/j.jcf.2020.07.014.

Sagel SD, Khan U, Heltshe SL, Clancy JP, Borowitz D, Gelfond D, Donaldson SH, Moran A, Ratjen F, Van Dalfsen JM, Rowe SM. Clinical effectiveness of Lumacaftor/Ivacaftor in patients with cystic fibrosis homozygous for F508del-CFTR. A clinical trial. Ann Am Thorac Soc 2021;18:75-83. doi: 10.1513/AnnalsATS.202002-144OC.

Sakiani S, Kleiner DE, Heller T, Koh C. Hepatic manifestations of cystic fibrosis. Clin Liver Dis. 2019;23:263-277. doi: 10.1016/j.cld.2018.12.008.

Salvatore D, Terlizzi V, Francalanci M, Taccetti G, Messore B, Biglia C, Pisi G, Calderazzo MA, Caloiero M, Pizzamiglio G, Majo F, Cresta F, Leonetti G, De Venuto D. Ivacaftor improves lung disease in patients with advanced CF carrying CFTR mutations that confer residual function. Respir Med 2020;171:106073. doi: 10.1016/j.rmed.2020.106073.

Sawicki GS, McKone EF, Pasta DJ, Millar SJ, Wagener JS, Johnson CA, Konstan MW. Sustained benefit from ivacaftor demonstrated by combining clinical trial and cystic fibrosis patient registry data. Am J Respir Crit Care Med 2015;192:836-42. doi: 10.1164/rccm.201503-0578OC.

Sawicki GS, Ren CL, Konstan MW, Millar SJ, Pasta DJ, Quittner AL; Investigators and Coordinators of the Epidemiologic Study of Cystic Fibrosis. Treatment complexity in cystic fibrosis: trends over time and associations with site-specific outcomes. J Cyst Fibros. 2013;12: 461-7. doi: 10.1016/j.jcf.2012.12.009.

Schneider EK, Huang JX, Carbone V, Baker M, Azad MA, Cooper MA, Li J, Velkov T. Drug-drug plasma protein binding interactions of ivacaftor. J Mol Recognit. 2015;28:339-48. doi: 10.1002/jmr.2447.

Schwarz C, Sutharsan S, Epaud R, Klingsberg RC, Fischer R, Rowe SM, Audhya PK, Ahluwalia N, You X, Ferro TJ, Duncan ME, Bruinsma BG. Tezacaftor/ivacaftor in people with cystic fibrosis who stopped lumacaftor/ivacaftor due to respiratory adverse events. J Cyst Fibros 2021;20: 228-33. doi: 10.1016/j.jcf.2020.06.001.

Secunda KE, Guimbellot JS, Jovanovic B, Heltshe SL, Sagel SD, Rowe SM, Jain M. Females with cystic fibrosis demonstrate a differential response profile to Ivacaftor compared with males. Am J Respir Crit Care Med 2020; 201:996-998. doi: 10.1164/rccm.201909-1845LE.

Sergeev V, Chou FY, Lam GY, Hamilton CM, Wilcox PG, Quon BS. The extrapulmonary effects of Cystic Fibrosis Transmembrane Conductance Regulator modulators in cystic fibrosis. Ann Am Thorac Soc 2020;17:147-154. doi: 10.1513/AnnalsATS.201909-671CME.

Sermet-Gaudelus I, Clancy JP, Nichols DP, Nick JA, De Boeck K, Solomon GM, Mall MA, Bolognese J, Bouisset F, den Hollander W, Paquette-Lamontagne N, Tomkinson N, Henig N, Elborn JS, Rowe SM. Antisense oligonucleotide eluforsen improves CFTR function in F508del cystic fibrosis. J Cyst Fibros 2019;18:536-42. doi: 10.1016/j.jcf.2018.10.015.

Shaughnessy CA, Zeitlin PL, Bratcher PE. Elexacaftor is a CFTR potentiator and acts synergistically with ivacaftor during acute and chronic treatment. Sci Rep. 2021;11: 19810. doi: 10.1038/s41598-021-99184-1.

Shaw M, Khan U, Clancy JP, Donaldson SH, Sagel SD, Rowe SM, Ratjen F; PROSPECT Investigators of the Cystic Fibrosis Foundation Therapeutics Development Network. Changes in LCI in F508del/F508del patients treated with lumacaftor/ivacaftor: Results from the prospect study. J Cyst Fibros 2020;19:931-933. doi: 10.1016/j.jcf.2020.05.010.

Sheikh SI, Long FR, McCoy KS, Johnson T, Ryan-Wenger NA, Hayes D Jr. Ivacaftor improves appearance of sinus disease on computerised tomography in cystic fibrosis patients with G551D mutation. Clin Otolaryngol 2015;40:16-21. doi: 10.1111/coa.12310.

Singh AK, Fan Y, Balut C, Alani S, Manelli AM, Swensen AM, Jia Y, Neelands TR, Vortherms TA, Liu B, Searle XB, Wang X, Gao W, Hwang TC, Ren HY, Cyr D, Kym PR, Conrath K, Tse C. Biological characterization of F508del CFTR protein processing by the CFTR corrector ABBV-2222/GLPG2222. J Pharmacol Exp Ther 2020;372:107-118. doi: 10.1124/jpet.119.261800.

Singh SB, McLearn-Montz AJ, Milavetz F, Gates LK, Fox C, Murry LT, Sabus A, Porterfield HS, Fischer AJ. Pathogen acquisition in patients with cystic fibrosis receiving ivacaftor or lumacaftor/ivacaftor. Pediatr Pulmonol 2019;54:1200-1208. doi: 10.1002/ppul.24341.

Smith NF, Figg WD, Sparreboom A. Role of the liver-specific transporters OATP1B1 and OATP1B3 in governing drug elimination. Expert Opin Drug Metab Toxicol. 2005;1:429-45. doi: 10.1517/17425255.1.3.429.

Sosnay PR, Siklosi KR, Van Goor F, Kaniecki K, Yu H, Sharma N, Ramalho AS, Amaral MD, Dorfman R, Zielenski J, Masica DL, Karchin R, Millen L, Thomas PJ, Patrinos GP, Corey M, Lewis MH, Rommens JM, Castellani C, Penland CM, Cutting GR. Defining the disease liability of variants in the cystic fibrosis transmembrane conductance regulator gene. Nat Genet. 2013;45:1160-7. doi: 10.1038/ng.2745.

Stallings VA, Sainath N, Oberle M, Bertolaso C, Schall JI. Energy balance and mechanisms of weight gain with Ivacaftor treatment of cystic fibrosis gating mutations. J Pediatr 2018;201:229-37.e4. doi: 10.1016/j.jpeds.2018.05.018

Stylemans D, Darquenne C, Schuermans D, Verbanck S, Vanderhelst E. Peripheral lung effect of elexacaftor/tezacaftor/ivacaftor in adult cystic fibrosis. J Cyst Fibros 2021:S1569-1993(21)00098-9. doi: 10.1016/j.jcf.2021.03.016.

Sun T, Sun Z, Jiang Y, Ferguson AA, Pilewski JM, Kolls JK, Chen W, Chen K. Transcriptomic responses to ivacaftor and prediction of Ivacaftor clinical responsiveness. Am J Respir Cell Mol Biol 2019 ;61: 643-52. doi: 10.1165/rcmb.2019-0032OC.

Sun X, Yi Y, Yan Z, Rosen BH, Liang B, Winter MC, Evans TIA, Rotti PG, Yang Y, Gray JS, Park SY, Zhou W, Zhang Y, Moll SR, Woody L, Tran DM, Jiang L, Vonk AM, Beekman JM, Negulescu P, Van Goor F, Fiorino DF, Gibson-Corley KN, Engelhardt JF. In utero and postnatal VX-770 administration rescues multiorgan disease in a ferret model of cystic fibrosis. Sci Transl Med 2019; 11:eaau7531. doi: 10.1126/scitranslmed.aau7531.

Sutharsan S, McKone EF, Downey DG, Duckers J, Mac Gregor G, Tullis E, Van Braeckel E, Wainwright CE, Watson D, Ahluwalia N, Bruinsma BG, Harris C, Lam AP, Lou Y, Moskowitz SM, Tian S, Yuan J, Waltz D, Mall MA; VX18-445-109 study group. Efficacy and safety of elexacaftor plus tezacaftor plus ivacaftor versus tezacaftor plus ivacaftor in people with cystic fibrosis homozygous for F508del-CFTR: a 24-week, multicentre, randomised, double-blind, active-controlled, phase 3b trial. Lancet Respir Med. 2021:S2213-2600(21)00454-9. doi: 10.1016/S2213-2600(21)00454-9.

Talamo Guevara M, McColley SA. The safety of lumacaftor and ivacaftor for the treatment of cystic fibrosis. Expert Opin Drug Saf. 2017;16:1305-1311. doi: 10.1080/14740338.2017.1372419.

Taylor-Cousar JL, Jain M, Barto TL, Haddad T, Atkinson J, Tian S, Tang R, Marigowda G, Waltz D, Pilewski J; VX14-809-106 Investigator Group. Lumacaftor/ivacaftor in patients with cystic fibrosis and advanced lung disease homozygous for F508del-CFTR. J Cyst Fibros 2018;17:228-235. doi: 10.1016/j.jcf.2017.09.012.

Taylor-Cousar JL, Munck A, McKone EF, van der Ent CK, Moeller A, Simard C, Wang LT, Ingenito EP, McKee C, Lu Y, Lekstrom-Himes J, Elborn JS. Tezacaftor-Ivacaftor in patients with cystic fibrosis homozygous for Phe508del. N Engl J Med 2017;377:2013-23. doi: 10.1056/NEJMoa1709846.

Taylor-Cousar J, Niknian M, Gilmartin G, Pilewski JM; VX11-770-901 investigators. Effect of ivacaftor in patients with advanced cystic fibrosis and a G551D-CFTR mutation: Safety and efficacy in an expanded access program in the United States. J Cyst Fibros 2016;15:116-22. doi: 10.1016/j.jcf.2015.01.008.

Taylor-Cousar JL, Jain R. Maternal and fetal outcomes following elexacaftor-tezacaftor-ivacaftor use during pregnancy and lactation. J Cyst Fibros 2021;20:402-406. doi: 10.1016/j.jcf.2021.03.006.

Thorat T, McGarry LJ, Jariwala-Parikh K, Limone B, Bonafede M, Chandarana K, Konstan MW. Long-term impact of Ivacaftor on healthcare resource utilization among people with cystic fibrosis in the United States. Pulm Ther 2021;7:281-293. doi: 10.1007/s41030-021-00154-9

Tong K, Barker D, France M, Burr L, Greville H, Visser S, Middleton P, Wainwright C, Dorahy D, Wark P. Lumacaftor/ivacaftor reduces exacerbations in adults homozygous for Phe508del mutation with severe lung disease. J Cyst Fibros 2020;19:415-20. doi: 10.1016/j.jcf.2019.12.006.

Trimble AT, Donaldson SH. Ivacaftor withdrawal syndrome in cystic fibrosis patients with the G551D mutation. J Cyst Fibros 2018;17:e13-e16. doi: 10.1016/j.jcf.2017.09.006.

Tsai A, Wu SP, Haseltine E, Kumar S, Moskowitz SM, Panorchan P, Shah K. Physiologically based pharmacokinetic modeling of CFTR modulation in people with cystic fibrosis transitioning from mono or dual regimens to triple-combination Elexacaftor/Tezacaftor/Ivacaftor. Pulm Ther. 2020;6:275-286. doi: 10.1007/s41030-020-00124-7.

van de Peppel IP, Doktorova M, Berkers G, de Jonge HR, Houwen RHJ, Verkade HJ, Jonker JW, Bodewes FAJA. Ivacaftor restores FGF19 regulated bile acid homeostasis in cystic fibrosis patients with an S1251N or a G551D gating mutation. J Cyst Fibros 2019;18:286-293. doi: 10.1016/j.jcf.2018.09.001.

Van der Plas SE, Kelgtermans H, Mammoliti O, Menet C, Tricarico G, De Blieck A, Joannesse C, De Munck T, Lambin D, Cowart M, Dropsit S, Martina SLX, Gees M, Wesse AS, Conrath K, Andrews M. Discovery of GLPG2451, a novel once daily potentiator for the treatment of cystic fibrosis. J Med Chem 2021;64:343-353. doi: 10.1021/acs.jmedchem.0c01796.

Van Goor F, Hadida S, Grootenhuis PD, Burton B, Cao D, Neuberger T, Turnbull A, Singh A, Joubran J, Hazlewood A, Zhou J, McCartney J, Arumugam V, Decker C, Yang J, Young C, Olson ER, Wine JJ, Frizzell RA, Ashlock M, Negulescu P. Rescue of CF airway epithelial cell function in vitro by a CFTR potentiator, VX-770. Proc Natl Acad Sci U S A. 2009;106:18825-30. doi: 10.1073/pnas.0904709106.

Van Goor F, Hadida S, Grootenhuis PD, Burton B, Stack JH, Straley KS, Decker CJ, Miller M, McCartney J, Olson ER, Wine JJ, Frizzell RA, Ashlock M, Negulescu PA. Correction of the F508del-CFTR protein processing defect in vitro by the investigational drug VX-809. Proc Natl Acad Sci U S A 2011; 108:18843-8. doi: 10.1073/pnas.1105787108.

Van Goor F, Yu H, Burton B, Hoffman BJ. Effect of ivacaftor on CFTR forms with missense mutations associated with defects in protein processing or function. J Cyst Fibros. 2014;13:29-36. doi: 10.1016/j.jcf.2013.06.008.

van Koningsbruggen-Rietschel S, Conrath K, Fischer R, Sutharsan S, Kempa A, Gleiber W, Schwarz C, Hector A, Van Osselaer N, Pano A, Corveleyn S, Bwirire D, Santermans E, Muller K, Bellaire S, Van de Steen O. GLPG2737 in lumacaftor/ivacaftor-treated CF subjects homozygous for the F508del mutation: A randomized phase 2A trial (PELICAN). J Cyst Fibros. 2020;19:292-298. doi: 10.1016/j.jcf.2019.09.006.

Veit G, Avramescu RG, Perdomo D, Phuan PW, Bagdany M, Apaja PM, Borot F, Szollosi D, Wu YS, Finkbeiner WE, Hegedus T, Verkman AS, Lukacs GL. Some gating potentiators, including VX-770, diminish ΔF508-CFTR functional expression. Sci Transl Med 2014;6:246ra97. doi: 10.1126/ scitranslmed.3008889.

Veit G, Oliver K, Apaja PM, Perdomo D, Bidaud-Meynard A, Lin ST, Guo J, Icyuz M, Sorscher EJ, Hartman JL IV, Lukacs GL. Ribosomal stalk protein silencing partially corrects the ΔF508-CFTR functional expression defect. PLoS Biol 2016;14:e1002462. doi: 10.1371/journal.pbio.1002462.

Veit G, Xu H, Dreano E, Avramescu RG, Bagdany M, Beitel LK, Roldan A, Hancock MA, Lay C, Li W, Morin K, Gao S, Mak PA, Ainscow E, Orth AP, McNamara P, Edelman A, Frenkiel S, Matouk E, Sermet-Gaudelus I,

Barnes WG, Lukacs GL. Structure-guided combination therapy to potently improve the function of mutant CFTRs. Nat Med 2018;24:1732-42. doi: 10.1038/s41591-018-0200-x.

Veit G, Roldan A, Hancock MA, Da Fonte DF, Xu H, Hussein M, Frenkiel S, Matouk E, Velkov T, Lukacs GL. Allosteric folding correction of F508del and rare CFTR mutants by elexacaftor-tezacaftor-ivacaftor (Trikafta) combination. JCI Insight 2020;5:e139983. doi: 10.1172/jci.insight.139983.

Veit G, Vaccarin C, Lukacs GL. Elexacaftor co-potentiates the activity of F508del and gating mutants of CFTR. J Cyst Fibros 2021;20:895-898. doi: 10.1016/j.jcf.2021.03.011.

Veltman M, De Sanctis JB, Stolarczyk M, Klymiuk N, Bähr A, Brouwer RW, Oole E, Shah J, Ozdian T, Liao J, Martini C, Radzioch D, Hanrahan JW, Scholte BJ. CFTR correctors and antioxidants partially normalize lipid imbalance but not abnormal basal inflammatory cytokine profile in CF bronchial epithelial cells. Front Physiol 2021;12:619442. doi: 10.3389/fphys.2021.619442.

Volkova N, Moy K, Evans J, Campbell D, Tian S, Simard C, Higgins M, Konstan MW, Sawicki GS, Elbert A, Charman SC, Marshall BC, Bilton D. Disease progression in patients with cystic fibrosis treated with ivacaftor: Data from national US and UK registries. J Cyst Fibros 2020; 19:68-79. doi: 10.1016/j.jcf.2019.05.015.

Vonk SEM, van der Meer-Vos M, Bos LDJ, Neerincx AH, Majoor CJ, Maitland-van der Zee AH, Mathôt RAA, Kemper EM; Amsterdam Mucociliary Clearance Disease (AMCD) research group. Quantitative method for the analysis of ivacaftor, hydroxymethyl ivacaftor, ivacaftor carboxylate, lumacaftor, and tezacaftor in plasma and sputum using liquid chromatography with tandem mass spectrometry and Its clinical applicability. Ther Drug Monit. 2021;43:555-563. doi: 10.1097/FTD.0000000000000829.

Wainwright CE, Elborn JS, Ramsey BW, Marigowda G, Huang X, Cipolli M, Colombo C, Davies JC, De Boeck K, Flume PA, Konstan MW, McColley SA, McCoy K, Mc Kone EF, Munck A, Ratjen F, Rowe SM, Waltz D, Boyle MP; TRAFFIC Study Group; TRANSPORT Study Group. Lumacaftor-Ivacaftor in patients with cystic fibrosis homozygous for Phe508del CFTR. N Engl J Med 2015;373:220-31. doi: 10.1056/NEJMoa1409547.

Walker S, Flume P, McNamara J, Solomon M, Chilvers M, Chmiel J, Harris RS, Haseltine E, Stiles D, Li C, Ahluwalia N, Zhou H, Owen CA, Sawicki G; VX15-661-113 Investigator Group. A phase 3 study of tezacaftor in combination with ivacaftor in children aged 6 through 11 years with cystic fibrosis. J Cyst Fibros 2019;18:708-13. doi: 10.1016/j.jcf.2019.06.009.

Wang X, Liu B, Searle X, Yeung C, Bogdan A, Greszler S, Singh A, Fan Y, Swensen AM, Vortherms T, Balut C, Jia Y, Desino K, Gao W, Yong H, Tse C, Kym P. Discovery of 4-[(2R,4R)-4-({[1-(2,2-Difluoro-1,3-benzodioxol-5-yl) cyclopropyl]carbonyl}amino)-7-(difluoromethoxy)-3,4-dihydro-2H-chromen-2-yl]benzoic Acid (ABBV/GLPG-2222), a potent Cystic Fibrosis Transmembrane Conductance Regulator (CFTR) corrector for the treatment of cystic fibrosis. J Med Chem 2018;61:1436-49. doi: 10.1021/acs.jmedchem.7b01339.

Wark PAB, Cookson K, Thiruchelvam T, Brannan J, Dorahy DJ. Lumacaftor/Ivacaftor improves exercise tolerance in patients with cystic fibrosis and severe airflow obstruction. BMC Pulm Med 2019;19: 106. doi: 10.1186/s12890-019-0866-y.

Wood ME, Smith DJ, Reid DW, Masel PJ, France MW, Bell SC. Ivacaftor in severe cystic fibrosis lung disease and a G551D mutation. Respirol Case Rep 2013;1:52-4. doi: 10.1002/rcr2.27.

Yu H, Burton B, Huang CJ, Worley J, Cao D, Johnson JP Jr, Urrutia A, Joubran J, Seepersaud S, Sussky K, Hoffman BJ, Van Goor F. Ivacaftor potentiation of multiple CFTR channels with gating mutations. J Cyst Fibros. 2012;11:237-45. doi: 10.1016/j.jcf.2011.12.005.

Zemanick ET, Taylor-Cousar JL, Davies J, Gibson RL, Mall MA, McKone EF, McNally P, Ramsey BW, Rayment JH, Rowe SM, Tullis E, Ahluwalia N, Chu C, Ho T, Moskowitz SM, Noel S, Tian S, Waltz D, Weinstock TG, Xuan F, Wainwright CE, McColley SA. A phase 3 open-label study of Elexacaftor/Tezacaftor/Ivacaftor in children 6 through 11 years of age with cystic fibrosis and at least one F508del allele. Am J Respir Crit Care Med 2021;203: 1522-32. doi: 10.1164/rccm.202102-0509OC.

Zeybel GL, Pearson JP, Krishnan A, Bourke SJ, Doe S, Anderson A, Faruqi S, Morice AH, Jones R, McDonnell M, Zeybel M, Dettmar PW, Brodlie M, Ward C. Ivacaftor and symptoms of extra-oesophageal reflux in patients with cystic fibrosis and G551D mutation. J Cyst Fibros 2017;16:124-131. doi: 10.1016/j.jcf.2016.07.004.

6. Perspectives on mutation-specific drug therapies for cystic fibrosis

Isabelle Sermet-Gaudelus

Advances in the field of therapies of cystic fibrosis (CF) that target the basic molecular defect and restore cystic fibrosis transmembrane regulator (CFTR) protein activity have created unprecedented opportunity to transform and improve the lives and prognosis of patients. This provides a strong rationale for the so-called CFTR modulators as the new backbone of care for patients with responsive disease.

Indeed, since the study with ivacaftor in 2002, CF therapy has entered a new therapeutic paradigm with the concept of use of therapies tailored to a patient's specific *CFTR* mutations (Accurso et al., 2010). *In vitro*, ivacaftor restored p.Gly551Asp CFTR opening probability by ~50%, as well as muco-ciliary clearance, a hallmark of CF disease. In patients, the effect upon lung function was impressively rapid, dose-dependent, and reversible, and correlated to endpoints of *in vivo* CFTR function such as sweat chloride and nasal potential difference, creating proof of concept for efficacy. Since then, continuous efforts in academic and industrial research provided the roadmap to efficiently correct the multiple defects of the p.Phe 508del protein, and numerous other mutated proteins.

> The perspective for CFTR therapy are now to
> - (i) increase effectiveness of current CFTR-directed therapeutics for maximum long-standing efficiency and optimal safety,
> - (ii) develop therapies irrespective of *CFTR* genotype,
> - (iii) implement a new model of care in healthier patients from birth and
> - (iv) provide these therapies to all people with cystic fibrosis and potentially beyond.

Increase effectiveness of current CFTR-directed therapeutics

The notion that the clinical benefit of CFTR modulators is related to the extent of functional correction of mutant CFTR is based on observational studies of the relationship between the residual level of CFTR chloride transport and the milder clinical phenotype (McCague et al., 2019). This concept has been corroborated by the correspondence between the level of CFTR correction *in vitro* by ivacaftor or elexacaftor/tezacaftor/ivacaftor combination, also called highly effective modulator therapy (HEMT), with an increase of up to 50 to 80% of wild type CFTR function, and the mean improvement in lung function (~15 % increase in the percentage of predicted forced expiratory volume in one second: ppFEV1) as compared with p.Phe508del homozygous patients treated with lumacaftor-ivacaftor (restoration of around 10-20% of CFTR function and mean 5 % increase improvement in lung function; Middleton et al., 2019). These data indicate that full restoration of CFTR function should remain the ultimate goal to achieve maximum clinical benefit. Within this framework, the search for a multidrug therapy, consisting of correctors and potentiators might also include CFTR amplifiers to increase the CFTR mRNA transcript substrate pool.

The observation that the change in ppFEV1 is the same for those patients homozygous or heterozygous for p.Phe508del indicates that the target of maximum clinical benefit in the lung is not achieved with current HEMT (Heijerman et al., 2019; Middleton et al., 2019). This may be due to the fact that the patients already had chronic lung disease with irreversible structural damage of the airways, which will continue to deteriorate as also suggested by more long term real life data with ivacaftor, which showed that the treatment slows the rate of loss of lung function, but does not stop disease progression (Sawicki et al., 2015).

To what extent HEMT can break the vicious cycle of chronic polymicrobial infection, inflammation, and tissue damage is totally unknown. During the first year of treatment, ivacaftor tends to show a rapid reduction in inflammation markers from the first weeks, together with a decrease in *Pseudomonas aeruginosa* abundance, but this seems to be followed by an unexplained rebound of *P. aeruginosa* whereas ppFEV1 decreases from the first week but does not parallel infection or inflammation evolution (Hisert et al., 2017). In fact, until now, most trials did not explore outcomes of infection. We need more studies to understand whether the impact on short-term inflammation and infection will change long-term clinical outcomes and potentially define indications of co-therapies targeted to specific features of CF lung disease to maximize benefit of HEMT.

Follow up of patients on HEMT will also bring information about clinical evolution and potential adaptation of those therapies. A subset of individuals given HEMT may not exhibit pronounced benefit or could experience side effects that limit the ability to tolerate a life-long treatment. From this point of view, impact of individual pharmacokinetics has not been evaluated, and their potential factors such as CYP450 enzymes polymorphisms, age, nutrition, or co-therapies. Others may "escape/desensitize" after having been highly responsive thus leading to modification, or change of HEMT. It may be that CFTR modulator regimen may change throughout the life span, with potential alternating therapies.

Develop therapies irrespective of *CFTR* genotype

More than 2000 variants in the *CFTR* gene have been described, but the functional consequences are not defined for many. The majority of these *CFTR* variants are rare, occurring in less than five patients each worldwide, and their mechanism is currently unknown.

Using this framework, the concept of "theratyping" rather than the "one-to-one genotyping" targeted mechanistic approach helped to overcome molecular complexity and unknowns and showed that modulator drugs restored CFTR function across a broad range of variants. Those patient-derived planar cultures that allow electrophysiological studies of CFTR chloride channel function, can be obtained from brushed nasal cells at any age, and there is also the possibility to generate airway epithelial-like cells from skin or blood cells with induced pluripotent stem cell technology. Three-dimensional organoid cultures of intestinal or nasal epithelial cells allow to evaluate CFTR-mediated fluid transport. However, although those preclinical models have shown reliable predictability for *in vitro* testing of CFTR modulator on specific mutation, the question remains whether this preclinical laboratory testing might be used as a tool for individualized medicine.

Indeed, we lack data for correlations at the individual patient level between correction in CFTR chloride transport in those model systems, clinical endpoints (ppFEV1) and CFTR biomarkers (sweat chloride, nasal potential difference [NPD], intestinal current measurement [ICM]). To define the use of these tools, we need "Genotype-phenotype" clinical trials, gathering patients with rare mutations, linking *in vitro* testing of response to therapy in these patient-derived models, with clinical efficacy in the given patients and most importantly with effect on CFTR biomarkers. These primary cultures also allow to assess other less explored functions of CFTR such as bicarbonate transport as well as recapitulate the proteomic patient-specific background which may impact the patient response. Whether these models may be applied to predict with sufficient accuracy *in vivo* responses of individual patients with the same genotype is unknown. If this is the case, these patient derived models will be instrumental for the individualized assignment of the best drug regimen for any patient and offer a pathway for implementation of personalized medicine (Pranke et al., 2019a).

Finally, around 10 to 15% of *CFTR* mutations are not currently addressed by CFTR modulators (splice site, premature truncation defects, large indels, and severe folding abnormalities). Premature termination codons might be addressed by translational read-through and severe splice mutations by antisense oligonucleotides as already done in Duchenne's muscular dystrophy and spinal muscular atrophy. CFTR mRNA replacement therapy, gene therapy, or gene editing should be a mutation-agnostic ultimate goal. However, for all these strategies, barriers remain, including efficacy of delivery (where *CFTR* must be delivered, both anatomically and at which respiratory cell type, including the recently discovered ionocytes), circumvention of innate defense, as well as checking for off-target events. Whether mRNA or gene repair might be feasible in other affected organs is also unknown. The ultimate goal for gene editing in CF would be to target and correct stem cells to repopulate the airways and restore function throughout the lifespan. As stem cells are not easy to target *in vivo*, cell-based therapies using *ex vivo* gene editing is the approach currently developed (Pranke et al., 2019b).

Implement a new model of care in healthier patients from birth

With HEMT, the aim to transform CF from a fatal disease to a treatable chronic non life-limiting condition is not a dream anymore. With the impressive efficiency of these drugs, we need now to identify to what extent symptomatic therapies can be discontinued, thus reducing the burden of care. Those patients who are less symptomatic will be less willing to come to the hospital, and video conferences coupled with home-based spirometry might replace in some cases direct clinic visits. We need to evaluate effectiveness and safety of telemedicine.

With more healthy patients, we also need more accurate biomarkers to discern subtle lung disease changes. Measurement of lung clearance index has proved sensitive in young children and adults with mild disease. Lung imaging by ultra-low dose CT and MRI imaging of the lungs also hold promise as quantitative outcome measures. It is yet not appreciated how CFTR modulators might affect extra-respiratory disease manifestations (diabetes, liver cirrhosis, osteoporosis, chronic rhino-sinusitis …). Conversely, prevalence of new long-term complications in older patients may emerge, such as obesity, cardio-vascular complications and gastrointestinal cancers.

A cornerstone of the future clinical use of CFTR modulators will be their long-term safety and tolerability. Although current CFTR modulators have so far shown adequate safety and tolerability profiles (for 10 years for ivacaftor and 5 years for lumacaftor-ivacaftor combination therapy), potential side-effects caused by the addition of elexacaftor such as liver toxicity as well as some immune-allergic observations may be a source of concern. Indeed, these small molecules are known to bind directly to CFTR but their potential to bind to other "off-target" proteins and to interfere with other cellular functions, has not been studied. Therefore, long-term safety monitoring by pharmacovigilance programs are crucial across patient age groups.

Indeed, if these medications prove safe, the aim is to implement those drugs from birth with the perspective to prevent onset of irreversible organ damage. This strategy is still not validated by all, based on the fact that quantification of the effectiveness of CFTR modulators in children younger than 6 years has not been rigorously clarified and there are still limited data on safety in this population.

There are however strong arguments for this aim: firstly, the lungs of babies with CF are structurally normal at birth. Secondly, CFTR dysfunction in the airways initiates from the first days/months of life a muco-inflammatory milieu giving rise to irreversible bronchiectasis. This also favors early infection with pathogens, which is one of the main contributory factors in disease evolution. Thirdly, these early changes are potentially reversible, providing a window of opportunity for early treatment (Shantikumar et al., 2020). Therefore, it might be hypothesized that early initiation of CFTR therapies in infants with CF from neonatal screening has potential to delay or even prevent irreversible damage to the lung. It might also limit damage to other organs such as the pancreas and liver. One might even suggest potential indication of *in utero* therapy for the CF foetus.

Indeed, this concept of "preventative CFTR modulator therapy" is supported by studies in the p.Gly551Asp ferret, in which *in utero* initiation of ivacaftor and postnatal continuation led to improved growth, survival, conservation of pancreatic exocrine and endocrine function, absence of Congenital Bilateral Atresia of Vas Deferens and prevented mucus accumulation in the lungs and their infection. Very importantly, withdrawal of ivacaftor triggered initiation of CF-like multiorgan disease in the growing ferrets (Sun et al., 2019).

These data strongly argue for accelerated clinical development in early infancy and point to the importance of life-long adherence to avoid reestablishment and progression of disease manifestations. Most importantly, this must be counterbalanced by rigorous evaluation of long-term safety of the developing infant and preschool children. It is mandatory to accumulate substantial data in this area, over the next few years, to convince the medical community and the authorities of the benefits of early intervention.

This extends to the foetus as well, as these modulator therapies considerably improve the CF patient's fertility. As a result, it is anticipated that

90 % of the CF women with childbearing potential should be eligible for HEMT and thus give birth to CF heterozygotes. Studies aiming to understand the potential impact of these modulators on foetal development are urgent.

Provide these therapies to all people with cystic fibrosis and beyond

The ultimate goal is to provide global access of highly effective, safe and mutation agnostic transformative therapies to all people with CF at a price also affordable in developing countries (Bell et al., 2020). Well-validated *in vitro* assays for predicting clinical improvement might help tailor the drug regimen for a given patient and facilitate regulatory approval for rare *CFTR* mutations. If introduced early enough, at a time when organ damage is reversible, this would be the pinnacle of achievement of these modifying drugs in CF.

Last but not the least, these efforts not only pave the path towards optimal therapeutic strategies for CF patients but might be applicable for disorders linked to CFTR dysfunction (Patel et al., 2020). This includes mono-organ CFTR related disorders, such as pancreatitis, bronchiectasis, chronic rhinosinusitis and severe nasal polyposis, as well as other genetic and non-genetic conditions characterized by CFTR dysfunction. For example, *CFTR* heterozygosity is more frequently encountered as a risk factor for asthma, allergic bronchopulmonary aspergillosis or sclerosing cholangitis. CFTR dysfunction can be acquired in chronic obstructive pulmonary disease, among which cigarette smoke exposure, toxic metals and downstream effects of neutrophil activation pathways are the main causative agents. Clinical trials testing CFTR modulators in COPD are beginning. If proved efficient, this widens future therapeutic horizons of HEMT, potentially targeting a global population beyond the confines of CF research.

6.1. References

Accurso FJ, Rowe SM, Clancy JP, Boyle MP, Dunitz JM, Durie PR, Sagel SD, Hornick DB, Konstan MW, Donaldson SH, Moss RB, Pilewski JM, Rubenstein RC, Uluer AZ, Aitken ML, Freedman SD, Rose LM, Mayer-Hamblett N, Dong Q, Zha J, Stone AJ, Olson ER, Ordoñez CL, Campbell PW, Ashlock MA, Ramsey BW. Effect of VX-770 in persons with cystic fibrosis and the G551D-CFTR mutation. N Engl J Med. 2010;363:1991-2003.

Bell SC, Mall MA, Gutierrez H, Macek M, Madge S, Davies JC, Burgel PR, Tullis E, Castaños C, Castellani C, Byrnes CA, Cathcart F, Chotirmall SH, Cosgriff R, Eichler I, Fajac I, Goss CH, Drevinek P, Farrell PM, Gravelle AM, Havermans T, Mayer-Hamblett N, Kashirskaya N, Kerem E, Mathew JL, McKone EF, Naehrlich L, Nasr SZ, Oates GR, O'Neill C, Pypops U, Raraigh KS, Rowe SM, Southern KW, Sivam S, Stephenson AL, Zampoli M, Ratjen F. The future of cystic fibrosis care: a global perspective. Lancet Respir Med 2020;8:65–124.

Heijerman HGM, McKone EF, Downey DG, Van Braeckel E, Rowe SM, Tullis E, Mall MA, Welter JJ, Ramsey BW, McKee CM, Marigowda G, Moskowitz SM, Waltz D, Sosnay PR, Simard C, Ahluwalia N, Xuan F, Zhang Y, Taylor-Cousar JL, McCoy KS; VX17-445-103 Trial Group.Efficacy and safety of the elexacaftor plus tezacaftor plus ivacaftor combination regimen in people with cystic fibrosis homozygous for the F508del mutation: a double-blind, randomised, phase 3 trial. Lancet 2019;394:1940-1948.

Hisert KB, Heltshe SL, Pope C, Jorth P, Wu X, Edwards RM, Radey M, Accurso FJ, Wolter DJ, Cooke G, Adam RJ, Carter S, Grogan B, Launspach JL, Donnelly SC, Gallagher CG, Bruce JE, Stoltz DA, Welsh MJ, Hoffman LR, McKone EF, Singh PK. Restoring Cystic Fibrosis Transmembrane Conductance Regulator function reduces airway bacteria and inflammation in people with cystic fibrosis and chronic lung infections. Am J Respir Crit Care Med 2017;195:1617-1628.

McCague AF, Raraigh KS, Pellicore MJ, Davis-Marcisak EF, Evans TA, Han ST, Lu Z, Joynt AT, Sharma N, Castellani C, Collaco JM, Corey M, Lewis MH, Penland CM, Rommens JM, Stephenson AL, Sosnay PR, Cutting GR. Correlating Cystic Fibrosis Transmembrane Conductance Regulator function with clinical features to inform precision treatment of cystic fibrosis. Am J Respir Crit Care Med 2019; 199 :1116–1126.

Middleton PG, Mall MA, Døevínek P, Lands LC, Mc Kone EF, Polineni D, Ramsey BW, Taylor-Cousar JL, Tullis E, Vermeulen F, Marigowda G, McKee CM, Moskowitz SM, Nair N, Savage J, Simard C, Tian S, Waltz D, Xuan F, Rowe SM, Jain R; VX17-445-102 Study Group. Elexacaftor-Tezacaftor-Ivacaftor for cystic fibrosis with a single Phe508del allele. N Engl J Med 2019;381:1809-1819.

Patel SD, Bono TR, Rowe SM, Solomon G. CFTR targeted therapies: recent advances in cystic fibrosis and possibilities in other diseases of the airways. Eur Respir Rev 2020;29:190068.

Pranke I, Hatton A, Masson A, Flament T, Le Bourgeois M, Chedevergne F, Bailly C, Urbach V, Hinzpeter A, Edelman A, Sermet-Gaudelus I. Might brushed nasal cells be a surrogate for CFTR Modulator clinical response? Am J Respir Crit Care Med 2019;199:123-26.

Pranke I, Golec A, Hinzpeter A, Edelman A, Sermet-Gaudelus I. Emerging therapeutic approaches for cystic fibrosis. From gene editing to personalized medicine. Front Pharmacol 2019;10:121.

Sawicki GS, McKone EF, Pasta DJ, Millar SJ, Wagener JS, Johnson CA, Konstan MW. Sustained benefit from ivacaftor demonstrated by combining clinical trial and cystic fibrosis patient registry data. Am J Respir Crit Care Med 2015;192:836-42.

Shanthikumar S, Stick SM, Ranganathan SC. Minimal structural lung disease in early life represents significant pathology. J Cyst Fibros 2021;20:e118-e120. doi: 10.1016 (j.jcf.2020.12.010.

Sun X, Yi Y, Yan Z, Rosen BH, Liang B, Winter MC, Evans TIA, Rotti PG, Yang Y, Gray JS, Park SY, Zhou W, Zhang Y, Moll SR, Woody L, Tran DM, Jiang L, Vonk AM, Beekman JM, Negulescu P, Van Goor F, Fiorino DF, Gibson-Corley KN, Engelhardt JF. In utero and postnatal VX-770 administration rescues multiorgan disease in a ferret model of cystic fibrosis. Sci Transl Med 2019; 11:eaau7531.

7. Abbreviations

Abbreviation	Meaning
ABC	ATP-binding cassette
ACMG	American College of Medical Genetics
ACS	Adult stem cells
ASL	Airway surface liquid
ASO	Antisense oligonucleotide
ATP	Adenosine triphosphate
BMI	Body Mass Index
CF	Cystic fibrosis
CFGAC	Cystic Fibrosis Genetic Analysis Consortium
CFTR	Cystic fibrosis transmembrane conductance regulator
CFTR-RD	CFTR related disorder
CT	Computed tomography
DMD	Duchenne muscular dystrophy
ELX	Elexacaftor
ENaC	Epithelial sodium channel
ER	Endoplasmic reticulum
FEV1	Forced expiratory volume in the first second
FIS	Forskolin-induced swelling
FRC	Functional residual capacity
GRASP	Golgi reassembly-stacking protein
HEMT	Highly effective modulator therapy
ICL	Intracellular loop
ICM	Intestinal current measurements
iPSC	Induced pluripotent stem cells
IVA	Ivacaftor
LCI	Lung clearance index
LUM	Lumacaftor
MBW	Multiple-breath washout
MCL	Mucus layer
MRI	Magnetic resonance imaging
MSD	Membrane-spanning domain
NBD	Nucleotide binding domain
NMD	Nonsense mediated decay
NPD	Nasal transepithelial potential difference
PCL	Periciliary layer
PKA	Protein kinase A
ppFEV1	Percentage of predicted FEV1
PREFUL	Phase-resolved functional lung (MRI)
PSC	Pluripotent stem cells
PTC	Premature termination codon
RD	Regulatory domain
rRNA	Ribosomal RNA
SLC26	Solute carrier 26
SMPC	Summary of product characteristics
SOP	Standard operating procedure
TEZ	Tezacaftor
TMD	Transmembrane domain
UPR	Unfolded protein response
VI	Ventilation inhomogeneity
WNK1	With-no-lysine kinase 1

Table 7.1: Selection of important abbreviations used in this textbook. Further abbreviations are explained either directly in the text or in table and figure legends.

Index